Calculation Skills: For Nursing, Midwifery & Healthcare Practitioners

Calculation Skills: For Nursing, Midwifery & Healthcare Practitioners

Katherine M.A. Rogers

With contributions by Meriel Hutton

 Open University Press

Open University Press
McGraw-Hill Education
8th Floor
338 Euston Road
London
NW1 3BH

email: enquiries@openup.co.uk
world wide web: www.mheducation.co.uk

and Two Penn Plaza, New York, NY 10121-2289, USA

First published 2017

A catalogue record of this book is available from the British Library

ISBN-13: 978-0-33-524329-7
ISBN-10: 0-33-524329-0

Library of Congress Cataloging-in-Publication Data
CIP data applied for

Typeset by Transforma Pvt. Ltd., Chennai, India

Fictitious names of companies, products, people, characters and/or data that may be used herein (in case studies or in examples) are not intended to represent any real individual, company, product or event.

Contents

List of figures and tables

Figures

Tables

Acknowledgements

I wish to thank Meriel Hutton for granting me permission to work with her original manuscript for *Essential Calculation Skills for Nurses, Midwives and Healthcare Practitioners* (2009) in developing this book. Hence this book uses material from Meriel Hutton's book and updates it, as well as using and adapting some material from *Nurses! Test Yourself in Essential Calculation Skills* (Rogers and Scott 2011), and I wish to thank William Scott who worked with me on that textbook.

My sincere gratitude and appreciation also goes to my editor Richard Townrow and all the team at McGraw-Hill Education and Open University Press for their help, support and patience throughout the writing of this book. I also wish to acknowledge the reviewers of the manuscript and in particular Karen Hudson for her very useful feedback.

Finally, thank you to my husband Conor and sons Rory and Jack for their endless patience and understanding while I was writing this book.

Publisher's acknowledgements

The author and the publishers wish to thank the following lecturers and teachers, who helped advise us in finalizing content and figures for this book:

Paula Groves, Anglia Ruskin University, UK

Patricia Howlett, Anglia Ruskin University, UK

Karen Hudson, University of Essex, UK

Ellen Kitson-Reynolds, University of Southampton, UK

Grace Manktelow, Anglia Ruskin University, UK

Wendy Wright, University of the West of Scotland, UK

We also wish to thank the following lecturers and teachers for their involvement in developing the SmartBook and the digital content within SmartBook and Connect:

Steph Garner, University of Hertfordshire, UK

Matthew Hartwell, University of Bournemouth, UK

Karen Hudson, University of Essex, UK

Ellen Kitson-Reynolds, University of Southampton, UK

Mohamed Mehbali, London South Bank University, UK

Catherine Redmond, University College Dublin, Ireland

William Scott, Letterkenny Institute of Technology, Ireland

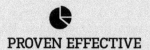

Mc Graw Hill Education connect®

McGraw-Hill Connect is a learning and teaching environment that improves student performance and outcomes whilst promoting engagement and comprehension of content.

You can utilize publisher-provided materials, or add your own content to design a complete course to help your students achieve higher outcomes.

PROVEN EFFECTIVE

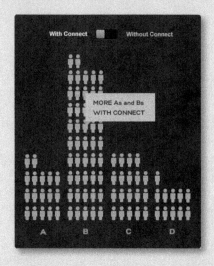

With Connect · Without Connect

MORE As and Bs WITH CONNECT

A   B   C   D

——INSTRUCTORS——

With McGraw-Hill Connect, instructors get:

- Simple **assignment management,** allowing you to spend more time teaching.
- **Auto-graded** assignments, quizzes and tests.
- **Detailed visual reporting** where students and section results can be viewed and analysed.
- Sophisticated **online testing** capability.
- A **filtering and reporting** function that allows you to easily assign and report on materials that are correlated to learning outcomes, topics, level of difficulty, and more. Reports can be accessed for individual students or the whole class, as well as offering the ability to drill into individual assignments, questions or categories.

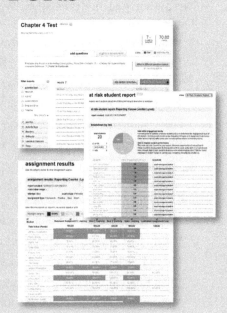

STUDENTS

With McGraw-Hill Connect, students get:

Assigned content
- Easy **online access** to homework, tests and quizzes.

- **Immediate feedback** and 24-hour tech support.

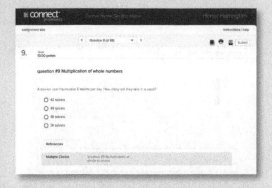

With McGraw-Hill SmartBook, students can:
- Take control of your own learning with a personalized and adaptive reading experience.

- Understand what you know and don't know; SmartBook takes you through the stages of reading and practice, prompting you to recharge your knowledge throughout the course for maximum retention.

- Achieve the most efficient and productive study time by adapting to what you do and don't know.

- Hone in on concepts you are most likely to forget, to ensure knowledge of key concepts is learnt and retained.

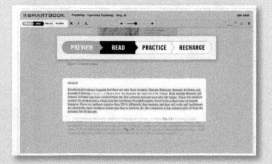

![Mc Graw Hill Education] **connect®**

FEATURES

Connect is an online assignment and assessment solution that offers a number of powerful tools and features that make managing assignments easier, so faculty can spend more time teaching. With Connect students can engage with their coursework anytime and anywhere, making the learning process more accessible and efficient.

SmartBook™

Fuelled by LearnSmart—the most widely used and intelligent adaptive learning resource—SmartBook is the first and only adaptive reading experience available today. Distinguishing what a student knows from what they don't, and honing in on concepts they are most likely to forget, SmartBook personalizes content for each student in a continuously adapting reading experience. Valuable reports provide instructors insight as to how students are progressing through textbook content, and are useful for shaping in-class time or assessment.

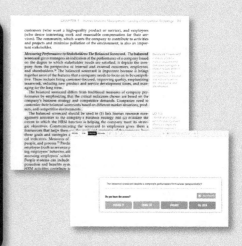

LearnSmart™

McGraw-Hill LearnSmart is an adaptive learning program that identifies what an individual student knows and doesn't know. LearnSmart's adaptive learning path helps students learn faster, study more efficiently, and retain more knowledge. Reports available for both students and instructors indicate where students need to study more and assess their success rate in retaining knowledge.

Introduction – how to use this book

This book has been written for students and healthcare practitioners who have to use and manipulate numbers in their clinical practice. The text is particularly suitable for all fields or professions within nursing, midwifery, health visiting, and operating department practice; it is also suitable as a primer for pharmacy students and non-medical prescribers.

Healthcare practitioners encounter numbers in a wide variety of situations during their practice. Some situations, such as calculating drug dosages, are more obvious than others; however, all require accuracy for the safety of the patient. As a healthcare practitioner, you need to be confident that you can deal competently with any numerical situation you come across, so this book aims to help you to gain confidence in your numeracy skills.

The book aims to provide an explanation for each type of calculation and outline a step-by-step method for working through the various types of calculations. Throughout this book there are **worked examples** to demonstrate the calculations. It is a good idea to practise the worked examples for each topic to enhance your skills and in preparation for the exercises in SmartBook. Where dates of birth are used, the annotation 20XX or 19XX has been used throughout the book to avoid 'dating' the examples.

Each chapter also contains boxes emphasizing **good practice points**, which highlight important concepts in numeracy and calculations that should help to improve your skills, making you a safe and competent practitioner.

This book introduces, on occasion, more than one method of doing calculations and it is important to recognize that other methods do exist. Practising different techniques can help you to learn what works best for you. Some useful formulae are given in Appendix D.

We hope you find this book a useful tool to conquer the essential skills required in your area of healthcare practice, and that you can return to the book whenever you need to revise your knowledge or to further your expertise.

Finally, in this book we have intended to minimize the number of references to guidelines produced by regulatory bodies for the various health professions. As this book is aimed at a range of professions it was not considered wise to include detailed guidance from nursing and midwifery boards or other specific professional bodies (such as the HCPC), especially when such guidance may change over time. It is however essential for all students and healthcare professionals to be aware of and understand the standards relevant to your profession, and to keep up to date with the guidance provided by the body governing your profession.

Part 1

Basic numeracy skills

1 The rules of basic calculations

This chapter covers:

- Basic mathematical operations: addition, subtraction, multiplication, and division
- Indices
- Order of operation: how to perform mixed calculations correctly

Introduction

This chapter reviews the fundamental mathematical concepts required for all types of calculations – from daily life to more complex numeracy operations required in certain areas of clinical practice.

Remember to practise the relevant **worked examples** outlined in this chapter to enhance your skills and in preparation for the exercises in the SmartBook.

Addition

Addition is the process of adding or combining numbers to find their sum. It is signified by the plus sign (+). It is also one of the most common types of calculation that we routinely use.

In clinical situations, addition may be used to determine the total number of tablets administered to a patient, or when calculating a National Early Warning Score (NEWS) chart.

Addition has a number of important traits:

- it is *commutative*, meaning that the order in which we add the numbers does not matter, thus changing the order will not change the result;
- it is *associative*, meaning that when adding more than two numbers, the order in which addition is performed does not matter.
- the addition of zero (0) does not change a number.

Table 1.1 shows the symbols and words used for addition.

Table 1.1 Words and symbols used to indicate addition

Word or symbol	Example
and	A 5 millilitre (mL) dose *and* a 5 mL dose is 10 mL
sum	The *sum* of three 5 mL measures is 15 mL
+	10 mL + 5 mL = 15 mL

 Good practice point

The National Early Warning Score (NEWS) is used to identify and respond to patients who present with or develop acute illness. It is based on a simple scoring system where a score is allocated to six physiological measurements already undertaken (and recorded on the clinical chart) when patients present to, or are being monitored in, hospital. The six measurements recorded are respiratory rate, oxygen saturations, temperature, systolic blood pressure, pulse rate, and level of consciousness. The scores are added together (adjustments may be required if a patient is receiving oxygen supplementation) and if the total exceeds a given threshold, this will trigger a clinical alert and response. NEWS charts should not be used in pregnancy, instead the Modified Early Obstetric Warning System (MEOWS) guidelines should be used. A separate chart also exists for child patients – the Paediatric Early Warning Score (PEWS).

Subtraction

Subtraction involves taking one number away from another to find the difference between them. Subtraction is represented by the minus sign (–) and you can see other symbols and words used in Table 1.2. Subtraction of zero (0) does not change a number.

In clinical practice, subtraction is used to calculate the difference between fluid input and output, over a period of time, in a fluid balance chart (FBC), or to calculate how long an infusion has been running.

Table 1.2 Words and symbols used to indicate subtraction

Word or symbol	Example
minus	Ten milligrams (mg) *minus* 5 mg is 5 mg
difference	The *difference* between 15 mg and 10 mg is 5 mg
–	10 mg – 5 mg = 5 mg

Multiplication

Multiplication can be defined as repeated addition. A number is added to itself, a specific number of times, forming a *product*:

$$2 \times 2 \times 2 = 8$$

The numbers that are multiplied to form the product are called the *factors*. Multiplication is represented by the symbol × and other words or symbols used are shown in Table 1.3. Multiplying any number by 1 does not change it; multiplying any number by zero (0) always results in a product (or answer) that equals 0.

In clinical practice, multiplication is used to calculate the number of tablets a patient should receive in a prescribed dose, or in other types of dosage calculations.

Table 1.3 Words and symbols used to indicate multiplication

Word or symbol	Example
of	Two *of* those 5 millilitre (mL) teaspoons is 10 mL
times	Two *times* a 5 mL teaspoonful is 10 mL
×	2 × 5 mL = 10 mL
*	2*5 mL = 10 mL
( )( )	(2)(5 mL) = 10 mL

Division

Division is the process of separating a given number into a specified quantity of equal parts. For example, if a person has a daily total of 50 milligrams (mg) of medicine to be taken in equal amounts twice a day, this means dividing 50 mg into 2 equal amounts, making 25 mg per dose.

In division, the result is known as the *quotient* (see Figure 1.1). The number that is divided is called the *dividend* and the number that divides it is called the *divisor*. Division is represented by the symbol ÷. Dividing any number by 1 does not change the number. Dividing by zero is 'undefined' and gives an 'error' message on a calculator or spreadsheet.

Figure 1.1 The components of division

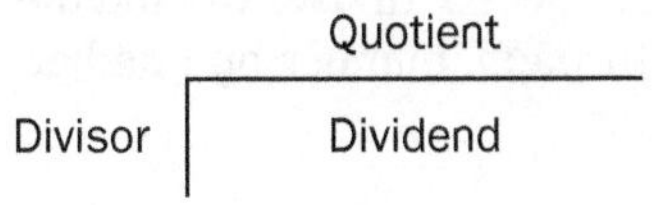

Quotient

Divisor | Dividend

In clinical practice, division is used to calculate the number of tablets or amount of a drug to be administered in divided doses, or the frequency with which a physiological event occurs over a period of time. Table 1.4 shows ways that a division can be written down.

Table 1.4 Words and symbols used to indicate division

Word or symbol	Example
over	50 mg *over* two doses = 25 mg per dose
/	50 mg/2 doses = 25 mg per dose
—	$\dfrac{50\ mg}{2\ doses}$ = 25 mg per dose
÷	50 mg ÷ 2 doses = 25 mg per dose
$\overline{\rceil}$	$2\overline{)50}^{\,25}$

Some division is easy to do in your head. For example, if there are 6 chocolates left in a box and 3 people to share with, how many can each person have?

$6 \div 3 = 2$

If you can not do the division in your head, then there are two ways of setting out the process to make it easier. One is called **short division** and the other is called **long division**.

Short division

Short division is used to find how many times a number will go into another when the *divisor* is small, but the *dividend* is relatively large.

Worked example 1.1: short division (producing a whole number)

You are part of a lottery syndicate with 6 colleagues. Your numbers come up and you win £372 to share between you. How much should each member get?

To calculate, you need to divide 372 into 6 equal parts:

$6\overline{)3\ 7\ 2}$

To divide 372 by 6, follow the steps below:

When setting up the division calculation, it is vital to get the divisor (6) and the dividend (372) in the correct place. Then divide through, number by number, starting from the left and working towards the right.

6 into 3 (or 3 divided by 6) 'won't go', so we put a zero above the 3 and try to divide 6 into 37 (or divide 37 by 6).

$$\begin{array}{r} 0\ 6\ 2 \\ \hline 6\,|\,3\ ^3 7\ ^1 2 \end{array}$$

From multiplication tables, we know that 6 × 6 is 36 and so we can put 6 on top of the bracket, above the 7.

The 1 left over from dividing 6 into 37 is carried forward to make the next dividend, 12. Since 6 into 12 goes exactly twice, we put a 2 above the 12. Thus,

$$372 \div 6 = 62$$

We can check that this is correct by multiplying back up:

$$62 \times 6 = 372$$

Good practice point

It is always advisable to check the accuracy of your division. This is easy to do – just multiply the answer (quotient) you get by the divisor. If the division calculation is correct, you should get your original dividend back (as indicated above).

Worked example 1.2: short division (producing a remainder)

Divide 516 by 5:

$$5\,|\,5\ 1\ 6$$

Follow the same steps as in **worked example 1.1** above:

$$\begin{array}{r} 1\ 0\ 3 \\ \hline 5\,|\,5\ 1\ ^1 6 \end{array}$$
Remainder 1

5 divides into 5 once, so we place a 1 above the bracket, over the 5. As there is nothing remaining from this part of the calculation, we then divide the next digit, 1, by 5.

5 will not go into 1, so put a zero above the 1 and carry it forward to make 16 the next number. 5 goes into 16 three times (5 × 3 = 15) with 1 left over. So we put a 3 over the 16 and comment that there is 1 remaining. Thus,

$$516 \div 5 = 103 \text{ remainder } 1$$

In this example, the division is not exact and there is 1 left over. We will deal with remainders later in this chapter.

Long division

Long division is used to help you find the answer to more complicated division, or when you do not know the multiplication table relating to the divisor. It is just the same as short division, but you carry out your calculation downwards, below the bar, so that the space directly under the bar does not get cramped with the large numbers remaining at each stage. It may be helpful to write out some times tables before working out the problem.

Worked example 1.3: long division

You move to a different hospital and join another lottery syndicate comprising all the theatre staff, a total of 63 people. Again (!), your numbers come up, and the syndicate wins a total of £34,524. We need to divide 34,524 into 63 equal parts, but we do not know the 63 times table.

First, set up the division in the same manner as for short division:

$$63\overline{)3\,4\,5\,2\,4}$$

Now divide. Long division is the same process as short division except that, because the numbers involved are bigger, your working is set out underneath as a 'subtraction sum' instead of using superscript numbers under the bracket. By writing down the result of multiplying the divisor by a suitable number, the subtraction sum (which in short division you did in your head) is set out for you, and the remainder to carry forward is provided automatically. Carefully follow the explanation to the left of the long-division sum set out below.

We can see that 63 will not go into 3 or 34, so we put a zero above those numbers at this point.

The 34 is now 'carried forward' to make the next number we need to consider, which is 345. The 345 can be divided by 63 a total of 5 times, giving an answer of 315 with a remainder.

Write 5 on the top line, above the bar next to the zeros, and write the product of 5 × 63 (315) under the 345.

```
      0 0 5 4 8
63 | 3 4 5 2 4
     3 1 5↓
     3 0 2
     2 5 2↓
     5 0 4
     5 0 4
     0 0 0
```

Subtract 315 from 345 to get a remainder of 30. Then bring down the next number (2) from the original dividend, keeping it directly below its position under the bracket (as indicated by the broken arrows above), and start dividing again. This time we are looking for how many times 63 will go into 302.

We can see that 5 times is too big and so we try 4 times. The 4 goes on the top line over the 2.

The product of 4 × 63 is 252, which we write underneath the 302, and subtract to get the remainder. This time it is 50.

When we bring down the last remaining number from the original dividend, in the same way as before, we get 504.

Now, 63 will go into 504 a total of 8 times and so we put an 8 on the top line and when we subtract the product of 8 × 63 (504) from 504 we are left with nothing, so the division calculation is complete. Thus,

£34,524 ÷ 63 = £548

Each member of the syndicate should receive £548.

Indices

An index number, or a power, is the small superscripted number that immediately follows a number or letter. The plural of 'index number' is *indices*. An index number shows how many times a number (or letter) has been multiplied by itself.

a^2 (read as '*a* squared') means $a \times a$. Here, a is multiplied by itself twice. The index number, or power, here is 2.

a^3 (read as '*a* cubed') means $a \times a \times a$. Here, a is multiplied by itself three times. The index number, or power, here is 3.

a^4 (read as '*a* to the power of 4') means $a \times a \times a \times a$. Here, a is multiplied by itself four times. The index number, or power, here is 4.

a^5 (read as '*a* to the power of 5') means $a \times a \times a \times a \times a$. Here, a is multiplied by itself five times … and so on.

[a^1 (read as '*a* to the power of 1') means '*a* multiplied by nothing else' and is therefore written as simply a.]

Any non-zero number (or letter) to the power of zero equals 1, therefore a^0 (read as '*a* to the power of zero') means the answer will be 1.

To multiply indices, add the powers together; thus $b^2 \times b^3 = b^5$

To divide indices, subtract the powers; thus $c^6 \div c^2 = c^4$

In healthcare, you may need to understand indices in order to interpret blood test results, or you may need this knowledge to understand the way certain measurements are recorded (see page 29).

Order of operations

Addition, subtraction, multiplication, and division are the four fundamental operations used in mathematical calculations. However, when doing calculations we are often faced with a mix of these operations, and so it is important to know the order in which we solve a mixed calculation because if we approach it in the wrong order, we can arrive at a very different (and incorrect!) answer.

The rule that is applied for performing calculations in the correct order is **B**rackets, **I**ndices, **D**ivision, **M**ultiplication, **A**ddition, **S**ubtraction (**BIDMAS**). To remember BIDMAS, use the mnemonic *Belly Itches Do Make A Scratch*.

Step 1: First, complete anything inside brackets. (*Note*: In the USA, brackets are called *parentheses*, so the letter 'B' becomes a 'P', which you may see in a slightly different mnemonic, so take care when using other resources.)

Step 2: Calculate any indices (or orders, powers).

Step 3: Work through any division and/or multiplication. Where there is both division and multiplication, work from left to right.

Step 4: Finally, complete any addition and/or subtraction. Where there is both addition and subtraction, work from left to right (as you read) or do all the addition followed by all the subtraction.

Worked example 1.4: order of operations

Calculate $7 + (6 \times 5^2 + 3)$.

To do this calculation, start inside the <u>B</u>rackets, and work out the <u>I</u>ndices first:

$5^2 = 25$

Therefore the calculation is:

$7 + (6 \times 25 + 3)$

Then <u>M</u>ultiply the relevant numbers inside the brackets:

$7 + (150 + 3)$

Then <u>A</u>dd the appropriate numbers inside the brackets:

$7 + (153)$

Now all the calculations inside the brackets are complete, we add the numbers outside the brackets to the value calculated inside the brackets:

$7 + 153$

Answer $= 160$

Chapter summary

This chapter has reviewed the basic mathematical concepts of addition, subtraction, multiplication, and division. A thorough knowledge and understanding of how to manipulate these key mathematical concepts is an essential skill in all aspects of healthcare practice. You should practise these calculations until you are confident in your ability to perform such numerical operations before progressing to more complex calculations.

2   Manipulating numbers: whole numbers

This chapter covers:

- Whole numbers
- Simplifying numbers that are fractions
- Unit conversions

Whole numbers

It is very important to be able to recognize number patterns and where numbers lie in order of magnitude. For example, recognizing that 1000 is 100 times bigger than 10, and 1000 times smaller than 1 million; or that 2.25 is smaller than 2.5, but bigger than 2.125.

It is unlikely that you will have to use this particular skill very often, as we often read large numbers out digit-by-digit, but it is still important that you can transcribe very large numbers accurately. Arranging in columns the digits which make up any number is a useful way of seeing the relationship between them, and keeping them in the correct order. You may remember at school writing numbers in columns, and this is a practice that will continue to be helpful whatever you are trying to calculate. It is particularly useful to keep strict columns when filling out fluid balance charts, especially complicated charts, such as those used in dialysis units.

In the table below, the number *five million, four hundred and twenty-five thousand, two hundred and ninety-four* is arranged in columns, showing how it should be written in digits:

Millions	Thousands			Hundreds	Tens	Units
	100,000	10,000	1000			
5	4	2	5	2	9	4

The thousands column can be subdivided into three columns. This is because it incorporates hundreds of thousands, tens of thousands, and units of thousands.

In the UK, it is conventional when writing a number in digits, to put a comma (,) after every three numbers, starting at the right-hand side, and so *five million, four hundred and twenty-five thousand, two hundred and ninety-four* looks like this:

5,425,294

However, it is also important to remember that using commas in this way is a convention not used in all countries. Many European countries do not use a comma and instead leave a slight gap, while in some countries the comma is used to signify a decimal point. Given these differences, it is vital that you use common sense regarding the magnitude of numbers, as well as carefully looking at what is written, especially when working with colleagues from other countries.

What about numbers that do not have a value for each column, such as: *one million, fifty-five thousand and six*? Where there are numbers missing from the columns, just put a zero. This can be known as a 'placeholder zero'.

Millions	Thousands			Hundreds	Tens	Units
	100,000	10,000	1000			
1	0	5	5	0	0	6

Hence, *one million, fifty-five thousand and six* looks like this:

1,055,006

Simplifying numbers that are fractions

Simplifying (or reducing) fractions means to express the fraction as simply as possible, for example, why say three-sixths $\left(\dfrac{3}{6}\right)$ when it means exactly the same (and is more easily understood) as a half $\left(\dfrac{1}{2}\right)$? Simplification involves reducing or cancelling down fractions and requires an understanding of *factors*.

Factors and the highest common factor

Factors are whole numbers that can be multiplied together to get another number. A number can have many factors, for example:

The factors of 12 are **1, 2, 3, 4, 6** and **12** . . .

. . . because **2 × 6** = 12, or **4 × 3** = 12, or **1 × 12** = 12.

When determining the factors for two different numbers – such as 12 and 30 – the **common factors** are the numbers that are found in both lists (*hint*, it is a good idea to write the numbers in a line across the page from smallest to largest):

The factors of 12 are **1, 2, 3, 4, 6** and **12**

The factors of 30 are **1, 2, 3, 5, 6, 10, 15** and **30**

The common factors of 12 and 30 are **1, 2, 3, 6**

The *highest (or greatest) common factor* is simply the **largest** of the common factors, so in the example above, the highest common factor between 12 and 30 is **6**.

Now that we have an understanding of what a factor is, the followings steps can be used to simplify (or reduce) a fraction to its simplest form:

> *Step 1*: Find the factors, i.e. the numbers that can be divided into the numerator and denominator.
>
> *Step 2*: Select the highest (or greatest) common factor, i.e. the biggest number that both the numerator and the denominator can be divided by. For example, for $\dfrac{5}{25}$ the highest common factor is 5.
>
> *Step 3*: Divide the numerator and the denominator by the highest common factor. This will give you the simplest fraction.

Lowest common denominator

Fractions are easier to manipulate if they are reduced to their *lowest common denominator*. When working with a number of fractions, the lowest common denominator is used for adding, subtracting and comparing fractions, rather than reducing each fraction to its simplest form. The lowest common denominator is often found through trial and error.

For example, when comparing $\dfrac{2}{18}, \dfrac{1}{3}$ and $\dfrac{4}{6}$, the lowest common denominator is 18 – so these fractions can be written as $\dfrac{2}{18}, \dfrac{6}{18}$ and $\dfrac{12}{18}$ respectively; using the lowest common denominator makes fractions easier to add, subtract or compare.

 Good practice point

There are some useful number patterns that help make calculations involving fractions a lot easier:

- Even numbers can be divided by 2, and in some cases by multiples of 2
- Numbers ending in 5 or 0 can be divided by 5

Unit conversions

The UK uses the metric system of measurement, which relies on decimals. It is a useful system because it simplifies the calculation of large and small units of measurement, and has been adopted by most countries of the world.

The basic units of measurement in this system include the metre (length [m]), litre (volume [L]), and weight (kilogram [kg]).

Multiples and subdivisions of these units are indicated by a prefix before the basic unit; for example, millilitre (mL) has the prefix 'milli' – and each prefix used in the system represents a multiple of 10 (see Table 2.1).

Table 2.1 Common metric prefixes

Prefix	Symbol	Multiple of 10
kilo	k	1000
hecto	h	100
deka	dk	10
deci	d	0.1 (1/10)
centi	c	0.01 (1/100)
milli	m	0.001 (1/1000)
micro	mc (μ)	0.000001 (1/1,000,000)

Since the metric system is based on decimals, it is quite simple to convert from one metric unit to another.

To convert a larger unit to a smaller unit, move the decimal point to the right and multiply by a multiple of 10.

To convert a smaller unit to a larger unit, move the decimal point to the left and divide by a multiple of 10.

There is a simple mnemonic to help with remembering the rules for conversion:

Mister Rabbit Died Laughing

Multiply Right, Divide Left

For example, take the conversion of millimetres to a larger unit, centimetres: 12 millimetres = 1.2 centimetres. As you can see, we moved the decimal in the number 12.0 to the left to get 1.2.

It is important to be familiar with converting between measurements, for example, in 2 grams there are 2000 milligrams, and in 0.25 grams there are 250 milligrams, and in 0.5 litres there are 500 millilitres.

In Figure 2.1 a ladder has been used as a visual way to illustrate unit conversions.

Figure 2.1 An illustration of unit conversions
Source: Karen Hudson, 2016. Adapted and reproduced with permission.

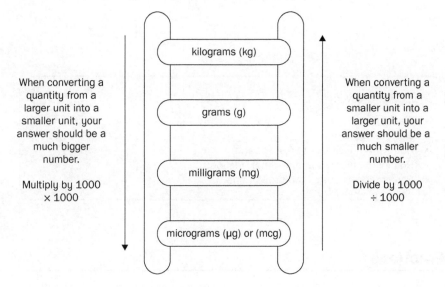

 Good practice point

Unit conversions are frequently used in drug calculations to determine drug doses. To prevent drug errors, it is always very important to double-check drug calculations that may require unit conversions.

Chapter summary

It is essential that all healthcare professionals are capable and confident in their ability to manipulate numbers because many drug errors are caused by human error through inaccurate calculation technique. Building on the basic numeracy skills covered in Chapter 1, this chapter has explained more about whole numbers, how to simplify fractions, and looked at some key units of measurement in the metric system. In the next chapter, we will learn more about using fractions and decimals as well as ratios and percentages.

3 Manipulating numbers: fractions, decimals, and percentages

This chapter covers:

- Fractions
- Decimal numbers
- Converting decimals to fractions
- Rounding numbers and decimal fractions
- Percentages, ratios, and proportions

Fractions

Parts of a whole number can be expressed either as fractions or using decimals. A fraction indicates that division is occurring; a fraction can be represented by any number, divided by any other number. The bottom number (the *denominator*) represents the total number of equal parts; the top number (the *numerator*) represents a certain number of parts out of this total; and the line between them indicates division.

$$\frac{numerator}{denominator}$$

For example:

1 hour is made up of 60 minutes (60 'parts').

$\frac{1}{2}$ an hour is one hour divided equally into 2 equal parts (of 30 minutes each).

$\frac{1}{4}$ of an hour is one hour divided into 4 equal parts (each part is 15 minutes).

So $\frac{3}{4}$ of an hour is 3 × 15 minutes = 45 minutes.

If the numerator is bigger than the denominator, it is called a *top-heavy fraction*. Simplifying a top-heavy fraction may result in a *mixed number* – a number that contains both a whole number and a fraction.

Improper fractions and mixed numbers

Improper fractions are fractions in which the numerator is greater than the denominator, such as $\frac{7}{4}$. They are commonly used in number calculations. An improper fraction can also be expressed as a mixed number (of whole numbers and fractions), which is an alternative way of presenting improper fractions. For instance, $\frac{7}{4}$ as a mixed number would be written $1\frac{3}{4}$. When doing calculations, it is often easier to work with improper fractions than mixed numbers.

Multiplying and dividing fractions

This is something that you will have to do regularly if you use a formula for drug dosage calculation, as well as when calculating drip rates for intravenous infusions (see Chapter 8) or parenteral nutrition in neonates (see Chapter 10). This section will explain the process in principle, using simple examples.

Worked example 3.1: multiplying fractions

The volume of fluid in half a cup, which when full holds 180 millilitres (mL), is half *of* 180, which is 90. This can be shown in fractions as:

$$\frac{1}{2} \times \frac{180}{1} = \frac{180}{2}$$

To multiply the fractions, multiply across the top row (numerators) to get 180 and multiply across the bottom row (denominators) to get 2.

The calculation could be simplified by cancelling down the original fractions. Simplification is possible when the denominator and numerator can be divided exactly by the same number (see Chapter 2). Thus:

$$\frac{1}{2} \times \frac{180}{1} = \frac{1}{2_1} \times \frac{\cancel{180}^{90}}{1} = 90$$

Dividing fractions is not often required in the calculations nurses have to make. The process is the same as multiplication of fractions except that the second fraction must be turned the other way up.

Look at the following example. We could say that to get half of 180, we need to divide by 2. This is exactly the same as multiplying by a half:

$$\frac{180}{1} \div \frac{2}{1} = \frac{180}{1} \times \frac{1}{2} = 90$$

Simplifying fractions

If we want to express 0.25 as a fraction, we need to simplify $\dfrac{25}{100}$:

$$\frac{25}{100} = \frac{\cancel{25}^{\,5}}{\cancel{100}_{\,20}} = \frac{5}{20}. \text{ And again} \frac{\cancel{5}^{\,1}}{\cancel{20}_{\,4}} = \frac{1}{4}$$

First, we divided both top and bottom by 5. The fraction is still not as simple as it could be, so we can divide again by 5 and reach our goal of $\dfrac{1}{4}$.

It is useful to recognize equivalent fractions and decimals that you will come across in healthcare. The shaded areas in the diagrams below show some common equivalents.

The shaded area is half of each shape and so all the fractions below are equivalent to a half or 0.5.

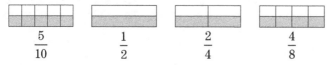

$$\frac{5}{10} \qquad \frac{1}{2} \qquad \frac{2}{4} \qquad \frac{4}{8}$$

In the same way, the fractions below are equivalent to 0.25.

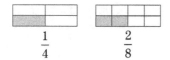

$$\frac{1}{4} \qquad \frac{2}{8}$$

Decimal fractions

Decimals are a way of writing fractions without using a numerator or denominator; instead, a decimal point (.) is used to distinguish between whole numbers and decimal fractions. Whole numbers appear to the left of the decimal point, and decimal fractions appear to the right. The value of an individual digit within a decimal number depends on its specific position in the number.

Each place to the left of the decimal point is greater than the previous one by a magnitude of 10. Each place to right of the decimal point is smaller than the previous one by a factor of 10.

$$1000 \quad 100 \quad 10 \quad 1 \quad \cdot \quad \frac{1}{10} \quad \frac{1}{10} \quad \frac{1}{1000}$$

$$\uparrow \quad \uparrow \quad \uparrow \quad \uparrow \qquad \uparrow \quad \uparrow \quad \uparrow$$

$$\qquad\qquad\qquad\qquad 0.1 \quad 0.01 \quad 0.001$$

In many ways, decimal fractions are easier to work with than conventional fractions, although it is sometimes necessary to convert between decimals and fractions.

A basic knowledge of this type of calculation is useful, since these types of numbers tend to be used interchangeably in clinical practice.

Addition and subtraction of decimals

Adding and subtracting decimals is not difficult if you keep to the discipline of lining up the decimal points.

Worked example 3.2: addition of decimals

Add 2.5 to 125.25 like this:

```
              2 . 5
  +   1   2   5 . 2   5
      1   2   7 . 7   5
```

If it makes it easier, you can add zeros beyond the digits on either side of the decimal point without changing the value but remember that they should not appear in the final answer.

```
      0   0   2 . 5   0
  +   1   2   5 . 2   5
      1   2   7 . 7   5
```

Worked example 3.3: subtraction of decimals

Do subtraction the same way. For example, subtract 65.75 from 124.8 as follows:

```
      1   2   4 . 8   0
  -   0   6   5 . 7   5
      0   5   9 . 0   5
```

 Good practice point

It is always good practice to approximate your answer before doing the calculation and to crosscheck afterwards.

When adding two numbers, you can check by subtracting one of them from your answer, which should give you the other number.

Thus, in the example above, if you subtract 2.5 from 127.75, you get 125.25. This confirms that you have added them correctly.

Similarly, after subtracting one number from another, by adding one of the original numbers to your answer, you will get the other original number.

Multiplying decimals

When multiplying decimals by 10, or multiples of 10, the decimal point can be moved to the right by as many spaces as there are zeros after the multiplier, resulting in a bigger number. For example, multiplying 48.1 by 10 results in 481.

Multiplying can be thought of as a fast way of adding, and we can check this by trying 6.5 × 10. Multiplying 6.5 by 10 is the same as adding 10 lots of 6 to 10 lots of 0.5:

$$(10 \times 6) + (10 \times 0.5)$$
$$= \quad 60 + 5$$
$$= \quad 65$$

which is what we would have got if we had simply moved the decimal point one place to the right: 6.5 → 65.

 Good practice point

A very common source of mistakes in nursing or healthcare calculations occurs when the decimal point is wrongly placed. A decimal point can be moved only when multiplying or dividing by 10, or multiples of 10. Always do an estimate, as this will help to prevent mistakes by giving you a guide to check against.

Worked example 3.4: multiplying decimals

Multiply 10 × 1.25. Estimate either by looking at it as an addition or by rounding the numbers to the nearest whole number: 10 × 1 = 10. Either way, our answer should be in the magnitude of 10.

Move the decimal place *one* space to the right as there is one zero in 10:

$$10 \times 1.25 = 12.5$$

Now check this against the estimate. The actual answer of 12.5 is in the same order of magnitude as our estimate of 10. Had our answer been 125 or 1.25, we would know immediately that the decimal point was in the wrong place.

Decimal numbers can be multiplied by whole numbers, or by decimals, in the same way as whole numbers are multiplied together. However, multiplying decimals requires an additional step to ensure that the same number of digits lies to the right of the decimal point in the answer, as in both the original numbers.

Worked example 3.5: multiplying decimals

A mother tells you she is giving her baby a 6.5 ounce bottle. What is this amount in millilitres (mL)?

You know that 1 fluid ounce is equal to 28.4 mL and so the calculation will be 6.5 × 28.4. Do a rough estimation by rounding the numbers to the nearest whole number, as this will help you place the decimal point correctly:

$7 \times 28 = 196$

Now set up the multiplication sum:

		2	8	.	4		
×			6	.	5		
	1	4	.	2	0		Row 1: multiply the top row (28.4) by 0.5
1	7	0	.	4	0		Row 2: multiply the top row by 6
1	8	4	.	6	0		Row 3: add together Row 1 and Row 2

Each of the two original numbers (28.4 and 6.5) has *one* number following the decimal point, so the answer (in Row 3) needs *two* numbers to the right of the decimal point.

$28.4 \times 6.5 = 184.60$

Check this against the estimate. Remember that having completed our calculation, we can drop the final zero to the right of the decimal point without changing the value of our answer. Thus, our final answer is 184.6 mL.

Dividing decimals

Dividing decimals by 10, or multiples of 10, is just the same as multiplying them, except that the decimal point moves to the left and the number becomes smaller.

Dividing decimals by other decimals is performed by changing the *divisor* (the number doing the dividing) into a whole number and then using the process of long or short division, keeping the decimal point in the same place for the answer.

Worked example 3.6: dividing decimals

A baby weighs 8.14 pounds (lb) and you want to know what this is in kilograms. There are 2.2 lb in 1 kg and so we need to divide 8.14 by 2.2 to convert from pounds to kilograms.

Estimate an answer first.

We can get a rough estimate by remembering that the same weight will be a higher number of pounds (lb) than kilograms (kg).

By rounding the numbers, we get 8 ÷ 2 = 4, and so our answer should be approximately 4.

Now calculate. As we saw earlier, a number divided by another can be written $\frac{10}{2}$, meaning 10 divided by 2. If we multiply both these numbers by the same number, the value of the answer will not change:

$$\text{Just as } \frac{10}{2} = 5, \frac{10 \times 4}{2 \times 4} \text{ and } \frac{40}{8} = 5.$$

Thus, to change the decimal divisor of our problem (2.2) to a whole number, the easiest thing is to multiply by 10 to get 22. We then have to do the same thing to the dividend (8.14) and we get 81.4.

So 8.14 ÷ 2.2 is the same as 81.4 ÷ 22.

We can now use long division, as we did with whole numbers, but keeping the decimal point in the same place:

```
        0  3  .  7
  22 │ 8  1  .  4
        6  6
        1  5     4
        1  5     4
        0  0     0
```

8.14 ÷ 2.2 = 3.7

By checking against the estimate, we can see that the decimal point is in the right place and our answer is 3.7 kg.

Worked example 3.7: dividing decimals

The shifts at your hospital last 7.5 hours each. How many shifts would you need to do to make up 1222 practice hours?

First, estimate using numbers to which you can easily relate. For example,

1400 ÷ 7 = 200

Next, change the decimal divisor into a whole number and change the dividend accordingly, i.e. multiply both by 10.

Now proceed with long division:

```
        0 0 1 6 2 . 9
   75 | 1 2 2 2 0 . 0
        7 5
        4 7 2
        4 5 0
          2 2 0
          1 5 0
            7 0 0
            6 7 5
              2 5
```

There comes a point with long division where the common sense of what you are doing should tell you to stop. In this instance, we are looking for a number of shifts and so we want a whole number. The answer we have reached (so far), if rounded up to the next whole number, will give us an answer of 163 and this is in the same area of magnitude as the estimate. Similarly, we can correct an answer to any number of decimal places by rounding up where the next number is 5 or above. Note that the decimal place did not need to be there when we began our division, but was put in when we ran out of numbers to bring down. In exactly the same way, the remainder in a division of whole numbers can be transformed into a decimal fraction.

Converting decimals to fractions

You may recognize *point two five* (written 0.25) as a commonly used decimal fraction, equivalent to $\frac{1}{4}$. How is 0.25 the same as $\frac{1}{4}$?

From the number columns (in Chapter 2), we know that 0.25 is the same as 25 hundredths or $\frac{25}{100}$. To turn 25 hundredths into quarters, we just need to simplify or cancel down the fraction, to reduce it to its simplest form.

Figure 3.1 An illustration using money

Source: Images provided under a Creative Commons Attribution-ShareAlike 4.0 International licence from Wikimedia Commons.

 =

As Figure 3.1 shows, five 20 pence coins makes £1.00, which means £0.20 is $\frac{1}{5}$ of £1.00. By removing the '£' symbol and the trailing zero, £0.20 becomes the decimal number 0.2.

Rounding numbers and decimal fractions

A decimal fraction describes a fraction where the denominator is a power of 10 (such as 10, 100, 1000, etc.), and because of this, decimal fractions can instead be written with a decimal point (and no denominator), making it easier to do calculations like addition and multiplication on fractions. For example:

- $\frac{6}{10}$ is a decimal fraction and it can be written as 0.6

- $\frac{39}{100}$ is a decimal fraction and it can be written as 0.39

- $\frac{74}{1000}$ is a decimal fraction and it can be written as 0.074

When calculating with decimal fractions, many of the smaller decimals to the right of the decimal point may become irrelevant, because they are very small in relation to the size of the overall number.

In this situation, the small decimal numbers need to be *rounded* to reduce the number of decimal places. There is a specific set of rules that apply when rounding decimal numbers.

First, determine the required number of decimal places to the right of the decimal point.

Second, if the digit to the right of the last of these decimal places is 4 or less, it is irrelevant and is ignored. For example, 5.46312 rounded to two decimal places would be 5.46.

Third, if the digit is 5 or more, then add 1 to the number to the left and remove the irrelevant digits to the right. For example, 5.46893 rounded to two decimal places would be 5.47.

In clinical situations, it may be useful to round numbers when dealing with weights or volumes that have a large number of decimal places. The amount of rounding needed depends on the level of accuracy required.

Percentages, ratios, and proportions

Per cent literally means 'per 100', so a percentage is a way of expressing a fraction as a proportion of 100. It is represented by the percentage (or per cent) sign, %. If expressed as a fraction, the denominator would be 100; when expressed as a decimal, a percentage has two decimal places.

To change a decimal to a percentage, move the decimal point two places to the right and add the per cent sign. In healthcare, percentage solutions usually refer to grams of solid dissolved in 100 mL of solution.

Sometimes drugs are packaged as a *ratio* or *proportion*, such as 1:1000 adrenaline. As manipulation of the numbers involved in such preparations is neither easy nor particularly common, calculations related to percentages, ratios, and proportions are dealt with in Chapter 10.

It is good to have a basic understanding at this stage of some examples of simple percentages you may encounter. For example, if you have 100 millilitres of 8.4% sodium bicarbonate, remember this is a proportion of 100, and so this means that the 100 mL solution you have contains 8.4 g of sodium bicarbonate. If you need to know how many grams of glucose are in a 100 mL bag of 50% (w/v) glucose, this is also simple: it is 50 grams.

You can change the following percentage strengths to ratio strengths:

50% =1 in 2
20% =1 in 5
0.5% = 1 in 200

Finally, to take an everyday example of a ratio, if you are making hot chocolate and the strength recommended is one heaped teaspoon per 175 mL and you have a 350 mL size mug, this means you need two heaped teaspoons for your mug to get the right strength.

Chapter summary

Manipulating fractions and decimals is a very common calculation performed routinely in most healthcare settings. It is therefore vital that all healthcare practitioners are extremely confident and proficient in performing such numerical operations.

4 Common measurements in healthcare practice

This chapter covers:

- Money management
- Time and the 24-hour clock
- Metric units
- Conversion between imperial measures and metric units
- Graphs

Money management

Many nurses, particularly those working in community and residential care homes, have to handle money as part of their role, whether it is keeping track of clients' own cash when shopping or taking into account the cost of individual drugs when prescribing medication. As part of their role, Ward Managers may be involved in budgeting and financial control for their wards.

The calculations concerned are not difficult but an effective system of keeping account of money gives clarity to patients or service users and their relatives and may protect you from being accused of dishonesty. Using a simple credit/debit account is useful for record keeping. This can be used with a running total (account style 1) or can be totalled at the end of the accounting period (account style 2) (see **worked example 4.1**).

Decimal coinage is treated in the same way as decimal fractions and just as with addition and subtraction, keeping figures in columns is recommended. Alternatively, printed accounts notebooks are available.

Worked example 4.1: weekly accounts

The care home where you work arranges for its residents to sell their craftwork through a retail outlet. Mrs Jones wishes to know how her funds are being accounted for and so you help her to set up a week per page record as illustrated below. This could equally be done for a monthly record depending on the frequency of transactions.

Note how, in **account style 1**, the balance is calculated each time there is an entry by adding figures in rows from the credit (paid in) column and subtracting from the debit (spent) column. At the end of December, Mrs Jones had £314.60 in her account.

Account style 1

Date	Item	Credit £	p	Debit £	p	Running balance £	p
	BALANCE brought forward from previous week, 31 Dec					3 1 4	6 0
3 Jan	Pension	8 7	9 8			4 0 2	5 8
4 Jan	Sale of work	1 2	4 0			4 1 4	9 8
5 Jan	Coffees			6	5 0	4 0 8	4 8
5 Jan	Papers			6	2 7	4 0 2	2 1
6 Jan	BALANCE to take forward to following week					**4 0 2**	**2 1**

In the second example, the balance is calculated at the end of the week by adding up the columns and then subtracting the total debit from the total credit.

Account style 2

Date	Item	Credit £	p	Debit £	p	Balance £	p
31 Dec	BALANCE brought forward					3 1 4	6 0
3 Jan	Pension	8 7	9 8				
4 Jan	Sale of work	1 2	4 0				
5 Jan	Coffees			6	5 0		
5 Jan	Papers			6	2 7		
Week total		1 0 0	3 8	1 2	7 7	8 7	6 1
6 Jan	BALANCE to take forward					4 0 2	2 1

Time and the 24-hour clock

In hospitals, it is vital that time is recorded accurately, such as in a fluid balance chart or when recording administration of drugs in a patient's chart. The 24-hour clock is usually, but not always, used to record time. This can be confusing and as with all numerical dealings, you must use common sense to interpret what you see.

Times using the 24-hour clock should be written as follows:

- 8 am = 08.00 hrs
- 12 noon = 12.00 hrs
- 8 pm = 20.00 hrs
- 12 midnight = 00.00 hrs

When calculating times, it is important to remember that although they look like decimal numbers, *they are not decimal fractions*; times are based on 60 minutes in one hour. Thus, when adding or subtracting times, we need to bear that in mind.

Metric units

The UK healthcare system uses the metric system, based on the Système International d'Unités (SI units), for most measurements. This incorporates metric units for mass (*gram*), length (*metre*), and volume (*litre*); these are the most common units that healthcare practitioners have to use. Larger and smaller quantities are given a prefix, which denotes whether they are 10, 100, 1000 or 1,000,000 times bigger or smaller than the basic unit. These prefixes can be applied to any of the metric units (see Table 4.1), but only the terms that you are likely to use as a healthcare practitioner are shown. In SI convention, the *kilogram* is the base unit of mass, but for the purposes of explaining relative size of units, here we will consider the gram as the starting point or 'basic unit' for measurement of mass.

Table 4.1 shows the relationship between the various measures. *Kilo* is used as a prefix for a value 1000 times the basic unit. One kilometre is 1000 metres. *Centi* is used to show that a measurement is one-hundredth of the basic unit. A metre

Table 4.1 Commonly used metric measurements and their relationship to the basic unit

Kilo	Basic unit	Centi	Milli	Micro	Nano
× 1000 (10^3)	× 1	× 0.01 (10^{-2})	× 0.001 (10^{-3})	× 0.000001 (10^{-6})	× 0.000000001 (10^{-9})
kilogram (kg)	gram (g)		milligram (mg)	microgram (mcg or µg)	nanogram (ng)
kilometre (km)	metre (m)	centimetre (cm)	millimetre (mm)	micrometre (micron)	
	litre (L)		millilitre (mL or ml)		

is made up of 100 centimetres. (You will come across the *centi* prefix in other situations – for example, centigrade, the scale used to measure temperature, centiles used in children's growth charts, and as a suffix in *percent*. 'Cent' always suggests that the number one hundred is involved.) *Milli* is used to denote 1000th of the basic unit. One millimetre is 0.001 or 1000th of a metre. *Micro* is even smaller and means a millionth of the basic unit. The diameter of a red blood cell is measured in microns.

Where very large or very small numbers are involved, the value may be expressed as 'a power of 10'. Earlier in this book we explained indices (on page 9) and so it should be clear what a power of 10 means. Showing a value to the power of 10 is a form of mathematical shorthand and indicates the number of multiplications or, in the case of negative power, divisions by ten required to reach the number. A kilogram could be written 10^3 g, indicating that it is 1 g multiplied by $10 \times 10 \times 10$, whereas a milligram could be written 10^{-3} g, the negative power indicating that it is *divided* by 10^3. A nanogram (10^{-9} g) is a tiny measure 1,000,000,000th of a gram and is used for a very small number of specific drugs.

Although the safest way to write a unit of measurement is in full, the abbreviations in Table 4.1 are generally acceptable. Note that it is strongly recommended in the British National Formulary (BNF) that microgram (mcg or μg) and nanogram (ng) are written *in full*, since their abbreviations are too similar to that of milligram (mg) to be safe. Although the full word may be written as a plural (e.g. milligrams), the abbreviation is not. Ten milligrams is expressed as 10 mg, *not* 10 mgs.

 Good practice point

Although the unit of millilitres is sometimes abbreviated as ml, in this book (and the corresponding SmartBook) we will use the mL notation because this is the abbreviation used in the British National Formulary (BNF) (and 'mL' limits confusion with the numeral '1' or upper-case 'i').

Occasionally, you may come across a prescription written for a drug using a different strength from that dispensed. For example, 0.5 g may be prescribed for a drug that is dispensed as 500 mg. You need to be able to calculate the correct strength before you can administer the drug to the patient. We can do this using an equation:

Worked example 4.2: converting between metric measures – grams to milligrams

0.5 g of a drug is prescribed. The label on the bottle states that each tablet is 500 mg.

Good practice point

Always convert the prescription to the strength of the preparation and not the other way round. So, we change the prescription (g) to mg.

Method 1. Remember that with an equation, as long as we do the same thing to both sides, the values remain equal.

We know that 1 g   = 1000 mg
So   0.5 g = 500 mg (both sides divided by 2)
                            = 1 tablet.

Method 2. We know that there are 1000 mg in a gram and so by multiplying 0.5 g by 1000, we will convert it into milligrams.

To multiply by 1000, move the decimal point three spaces to the right (one per zero):

0.5 g = 500 mg
       = 1 tablet.

Check that this is a sensible answer. Each tablet contains 500 mg and giving one tablet would be appropriate.

Worked example 4.3: converting between metric measures – micrograms to milligrams

A prescription is for 2000 micrograms. The bottle is labelled as 1 mg per tablet. So, we need to change the prescribed dose to milligrams (mg).

Method 1
1000 micrograms = 1 mg = 1 tablet
2000 micrograms = 2 mg (both sides multiplied by 2) = 2 tablets.

Method 2. Change the micrograms to milligrams by dividing by 1000 (move the decimal point three places to the left):
2000.0 microgram = 2 mg
Each tablet is 1 mg, so we need 2 tablets.

In medicines management, you will come across a variety of measurements of weight and volume. Occasionally, the term cubic centimetre (cc) may be used instead of millilitre (mL), particularly when referring to size of syringes, and these measures are used interchangeably. In other words, a 10 cc syringe is the same as a 10 mL syringe.

Drugs may also be dispensed in strengths other than the usual metric measures. For example, some hormones (such as insulin and oxytocin) are measured in units of activity and the prescription will be in a number of units (u). Sometimes these are termed international units (iu).

 Good practice point

Human insulin is measured in international units. When using insulin, it is essential that you use the correct insulin syringe, graduated in units (iu), not in millilitres (mL), when drawing up insulin injections. The safety of the patient is at risk if you fail to do so. This is because international units are not the same as millilitres.

Other metric units, which you may come across but are unlikely to use in any calculations, include:

- *Moles* (mol) and *millimoles* (mmol), which are applied to the molecular weight of chemicals and seen in laboratory reports.
- *Joules* (J), which constitute a measure of energy referred to in defibrillator use.

Although the metric unit for pressure is the *Pascal* (Pa), the most common measurement of pressure in healthcare is millimetres (mm) of mercury (Hg), which is used when measuring arterial blood pressure (BP) and central venous pressure (CVP), although CVP is occasionally measured in centimetres (cm) of water (H_2O).

Conversion between imperial measures and metric units (and vice versa)

Although the healthcare professions use metric units to measure weight and length, the traditional announcement of a new baby usually includes a weight in the old imperial measures of pounds and ounces and often a length in inches. Many people in the UK have been slow to incorporate the metric system when referring to their own height and weight and so healthcare workers need to be able to convert these units from imperial to metric (and vice versa). Although conversion charts exist, these may not always be at hand and so knowing how to do the conversion is useful. Converting between metric and imperial measures involves calculations that use several of the basic mathematical skills covered in Chapter 3, particularly calculating using decimal fractions. To be able to convert, you also need to know how many imperial units there are in a metric unit and vice versa. Here are some useful accepted equivalents:

- 1 kg = 2.2 lb (there are 16 oz in 1 pound and 14 pounds in 1 stone)
- 1 metre = 39 inches (12 inches in 1 foot)
- 1 fluid ounce = 28.4 millilitres.

Conversion is a key skill in a variety of situations, and one important area is in infant feeding, which is explained in **worked example 4.5.**

Worked example 4.4: converting kilograms to pounds and ounces

A newborn's weight is 3.45 kg. What is this in pounds and ounces?

First, approximate or estimate by rounding up or down:

1 kg is approximately 2 lb and 3.45 is nearly 3.5 or $3\frac{1}{2}$

So 3.5 kg will be approximately $3\frac{1}{2} \times 2 = 7$ lb.

Now do the actual calculation:

1 kg = 2.2 lb

3.45 kg = 2.2 × 3.45 lb.

(To multiply two decimals, go to Chapter 3.)

The answer you should get is 7.59 lb. But we have not yet got an amount in pounds *and ounces*. There are 16 oz in a pound and so again make an approximation:

0.59 is just over half and so our answer should be just over half a pound or 8 oz.

Now do the calculation:

0.59 of 16 oz = 0.59 × 16

= 9.44 oz, which is just over 8 and so is a sensible answer.

So our converted weight is 7 lb 9.44 oz.

As we do not use anything smaller than an ounce when weighing babies using imperial measures, the 0.44 can be rounded down and the nearest equivalent weight to 3.45 kg given as 7 lb 9 oz.

Worked example 4.5: converting fluid ounces to millilitres

Infant feeding is another area where lay people often use the imperial unit (fluid ounces) of measurement whereas the hospital is likely to use metric units (millilitres), particularly if the child is being tube fed. To get a good idea of what an infant's normal intake is, you may need to convert a mother's reported '7 ounce bottle' into millilitres (mL). Can you calculate this and round up the total appropriately?

To convert from fluid ounces to millilitres:

1 fluid ounce = 28.4 millilitres

So 7 fluid ounces = 7 × 28.4 mL.

This gives us 198.8 mL, or approximately 200 mL.

Note: We accept a rounding up of just over a millilitre in this case, whereas this would not be acceptable if we were dealing with much smaller amounts, especially if it involved drugs.

Graphs

The most common type of graph used in everyday healthcare practice is modified line graphs. These are used in nursing and midwifery practice to plot changes in a patient's condition, as on a patient's observation chart, or to compare measurements with normal values, as in a children's growth chart.

Line graphs are arranged on two intersecting (horizontal and vertical crossing) axes with independent scales (x = horizontal against y = vertical). For example, temperature can be plotted against time or changes in weight against calorific intake. The observation chart shows changes in the patient's condition over time and can be helpful in identifying not only the presence of fever (a high temperature) but the nature of the possible underlying infection. For example, some infections cause a higher temperature in the evening. The observation chart can also indicate the effectiveness of medication given to reduce blood pressure, bring down the temperature or steady a rapid pulse rate. Hence, understanding what the lines on the graph mean, and accurate plotting of a measurement on the chart, are important.

Figures 4.1 to 4.3 show children's growth charts for different sexes and ages and a symphysis-fundal height chart, used in midwifery. These charts are also called centile charts for reasons that will become apparent.

This type of graph is useful for plotting changing parameters, such as a child's weight or height, over time. A children's growth chart can be consulted to gauge whether a child is growing too slowly or too quickly compared with accepted norms. If a measure, such as height, is on the 2nd centile, this means that for every 100 children of that age, 2 (2%) would be expected to be shorter and 98 (98%) would be expected to be taller. This is not indicative of normality or otherwise from a single reading, but plotting a particular child's height and/or weight over time can be a useful indicator of health. In midwifery practice, the symphysis-fundal height chart may be used to help plot the growth of the foetus.

Figure 4.1 Girls' UK growth chart, 2–8 years

Source: RCPCH (2012). Reproduced with permission of the Royal College of Paediatrics and Child Health

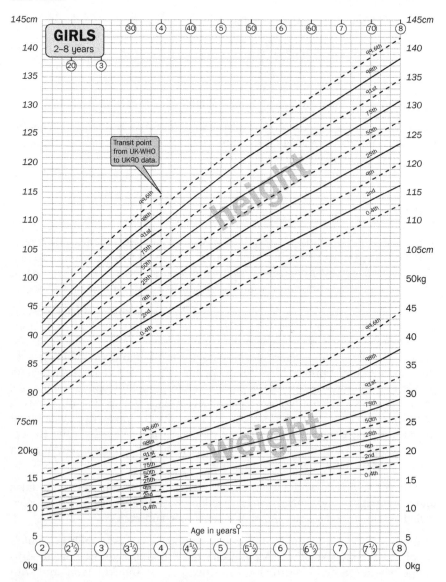

Worked example 4.6: using growth charts

To assess a female child of 5 years whose weight is 20 kg, we look at the relevant chart shown in Figure 4.1 to see where the 5-year line intersects with the 20 kg line. This is exactly on the 75th centile as marked on this chart, which

Figure 4.2 Symphysis-fundal height chart

Source: Reproduced with permission of the Royal Wolverhampton NHS Trust

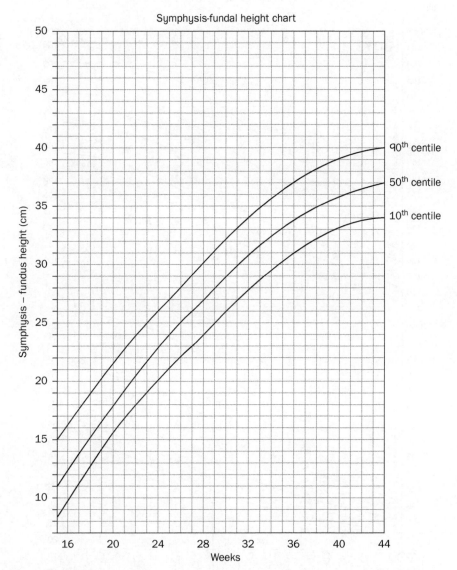

means that for every 100 female children at 5 years of age, 25 are likely to weigh more than 20 kg and 75 will weigh 20 kg or less than 20 kg.

If we assessed the same child at $6\frac{1}{2}$ years, we could expect her weight to be on the same centile, which would mean that at $6\frac{1}{2}$ years she should weigh about 24 kg.

Figure 4.3 Boys' UK growth chart, 9–18 years

Source: RCPCH (2012). Reproduced with permission of the Royal College of Paediatrics and Child Health

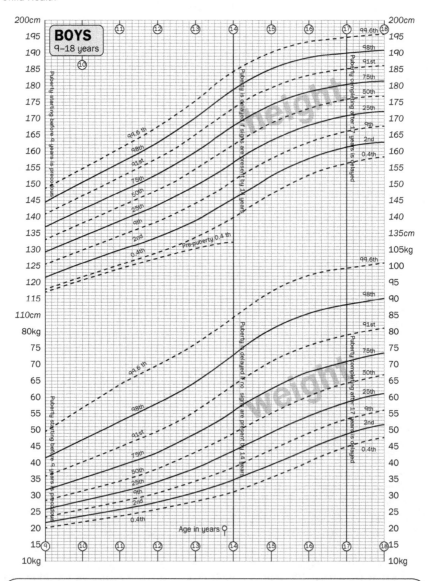

> **Chapter summary**
>
> The measurements explored in this chapter are typical of those used across healthcare practice. The following chapters cover medication and fluid prescriptions, where some of these measurements are used in different ways.

Part 2

Medications safety

5 Importance of calculation skills for safe administration of medicines

This chapter covers:

- Professional standards for management and administration of medicines
- Medication errors

All healthcare practitioners need to be able to use numbers with confidence, to ensure the safety of their patients, particularly when administering medicines. Entrants to healthcare courses must have good literacy and numeracy skills to be able to undertake the academic and practical components of their chosen course at university. For example, in UK nursing and midwifery, the specific guidance from the Nursing and Midwifery Council (NMC) relating to numeracy requires pre-registration students to demonstrate an ability to accurately manipulate numbers when applied to volume, weight, and length. It also suggests that this should include skills in addition, subtraction, division, multiplication, the use of decimals, fractions and percentages, and the use of a calculator. As outlined in the introduction to this book, you need to be aware if a professional body governs your profession and what the expected standards are.

Professional standards for management and administration of medicines

In the UK, the NMC publishes standards for safe practice in the management and administration of medicines by registered nurses, midwives, and specialist community public health nurses. Periodically these standards are revised and updated, so it is essential that all students and registered nurses and midwives are aware of the current standards, as failure to comply with the NMC Standards can affect patient safety and wellbeing, and risk a practitioner's professional registration (or a student's future registration). A registered nurse or midwife must check all drug calculations by nursing or midwifery students prior to administration.

Double-checking

The NMC recommends 'double-checking' all complex calculations. The process of double-checking (or second checking) involves each registered nurse (or midwife) doing the calculation separately and then comparing the outcomes. Once the calculation is cross-checked and agreed, it is important to consider the value in the clinical context – from your clinical knowledge, does the answer makes sense? For example, is the answer an appropriate volume for the prescribed medicine, the administration route, or the age of the patient? This double-checking is a good habit for all healthcare practitioners to use in practice.

Medication errors

Reasons for medication errors

Medication errors can have serious repercussions for patient safety and wellbeing. The majority of medication errors can usually be attributed to one of three types of human error:

(1)   the wrong medication being administered;
(2)   missed or delayed administration of medication; or
(3)   administration of the wrong dose of drug – which is most frequently due to calculation error.

This book will help you to reduce your risk of being involved in cases of medication errors, by outlining the mathematical concepts relevant to clinical situations and guiding you in practising your numeracy and calculation skills. Regular practice should help to improve your numeracy skills and make you more confident in your ability to apply mathematical concepts when performing calculations in the clinical setting.

Professional consequences of a medication error

Unfortunately, the media continues to report tragic cases of patient death caused by medication errors. In such cases, the fatal mistake(s) may be identified and reported during a Coroner's inquest into the patient's death. If a nurse or midwife is involved he or she may also be the subject of an NMC misconduct hearing into his or her actions that led to the patient's death. The outcome of a professional misconduct hearing will consider the details of the specific case, and determine the nurse's, or midwife's, fitness to practise. The NMC defines 'fitness to practise' as a registrant's suitability to remain on the register without restriction.

All healthcare professionals can minimize the incidence of medication errors by (1) having a thorough understanding of basic mathematical concepts, (2) being fully competent in their numeracy skills (outlined in Part 1 of this book, 'Basic Numeracy Skills'), and (3) regularly practising calculations, particularly those relevant to their area of practice (Parts 2 and 3 of this book).

Consequences for nurses, midwives, and healthcare professionals involved in medication errors

Case example 5.1

In 2016, an NMC misconduct hearing ruled that a Registered Nurse's fitness to practise was impaired, after she failed to adhere to a prescription when she incorrectly administered a drug that was prescribed for administration over 24 hours. In this case, the fitness to practise of the registered nurse who acted as the 'second checker' for the administration of the drug was not considered to be impaired, even though she admitted her failure to adequately check the medication prior to administration.

[Adapted from the 'Hearings and sanctions' section of the NMC website (accessed August 2016), with information from the BBC website www.bbc.co.uk (accessed August 2016).]

This case highlights the importance of understanding a prescription, and the procedure for accurate calculation of the drug dose to be administered over a specified time. It also emphasizes the importance of accurate and thorough double-checking. Each nurse or midwife is accountable for their own actions and has an important role to play in the accurate calculation and safe administration of the medicine. Furthermore, despite the distractions of a busy ward environment, everyone involved in the calculation and administration of medicines should give all steps in the process their full attention when undertaking such complex calculations and double-checking. By adopting these suggestions for good practice, you can minimize the chance of medication errors.

 Good practice point

For safe administration of medicines, always consider the following:

- Understand the prescription
- Understand the basic mathematical concepts required for the calculation
- Know how to perform the numeracy manipulation needed in the calculation
- Where possible, and **always** if you have any doubt about your answer, ask a colleague to 'double-check' your calculation
- Consider whether your answer is clinically appropriate
- Practise calculations regularly, ideally using practice-related examples

Chapter summary

To reduce the risk of medication errors, it is imperative that nurses, midwives, and all healthcare professionals are confident in all basic calculation skills before attempting more complex calculations. Generally, the more steps in a calculation, the greater the risk of error, so it is important to concentrate at all times when doing calculations. Remember to check your workings and double-check with colleagues.

6

Medications safety: administering tablets and capsules

This chapter covers:

- Prescriptions
- The importance of estimation
- Different ways to calculate medication dosage
- Formulae – how to construct and use them
- Checking your calculation

Prescriptions

One of the most common calculations that a nurse or midwife has to do is to work out the correct medication to administer from a prescription. There are several important elements to this skill, only one of which is the actual calculation. You have already learnt how to convert prescriptions from one unit of measurement to another and have done some basic calculations. However, the aim of this book is to help you with the calculation side of medicines management, which is what this chapter will cover.

When preparing to work out a medication dose, the first thing is to make sure that you understand the prescription and extract the information essential for your calculation.

Let's look at the fundamental information on any prescription – either a prescriber's pad (Figure 6.1) or a purpose-made hospital prescription sheet (Figure 6.2).

When calculating a drug dosage, there are a number of points you must consider:

Step 1 – Check the relevant information on the prescription:

- Name of the drug
- Format of the drug and route of administration
- Drug strength (*clarify whether the unit of measurement is the same on the drug packaging as on the prescription*);

Figure 6.1 Example of a prescription on a prescriber's pad

Pharmacy stamp	Age: 1 year 11 months Date of birth 4/6/20XX	Title, forename, surname & address Miss Lucy Patient 12 Anyold Street Hopetown
Number of days' treatment NB Ensure dose is stated	5	HO4 5PE
Endorsements	Amoxicillin oral suspension 250 mg/5 ml sugar-free 250 mg three times daily Supply 100 ml (No more items on this prescription)	
Signature of prescriber *Michael Dogood*	Date 02/05/20XX	
For dispenser No. of Prescriptions on form	Anyborough Health Authority Dr. M. Dogood 123 High Street Hopetown HO1 2PZ Tel: 0111 222 233	
		XXXXXXXX

- The time period over which it is to be given. Note that the way this is written will vary from place to place. Although explicit directions in English are recommended, some prescribers still use Latin abbreviations such as 'a.c.' for 'ante cibum' (before food). These can be found in Appendix A.

Step 2 – Look at the *label* on the medicine container and extract the information that you need to work out what you have to give. Information found on the label includes:

- Name of the drug (usually generic but may be a trade name)
- Dose per tablet/capsule/caplet
- Number of items in the pack (pre-packed medicines only)
- Expiry date.

Figure 6.2 Pages from a typical hospital drug chart

Hosp no. xxxxxxx D.O.B. 11/02/1978	SAINT SUNDAY Health
Surname Patient	HOSPITAL Service
First names Kevin John	Ward: 12
Adderss 12, Anyold Street,	Consultant: Mr. Surgeon
Hopetown,	Chart number: 1 of X
HO4 5PE	Number of charts in use: 1
	Other charts in use (please state):
	Drug chart re written by:
	Date: Checked by:

PRESCRIPTION CHART

ALLERGIES and DRUG SENSITIVITIES:	Type of reaction (eg rash):	Patient's own drugs:
Elastoplast		

Height 195cm	Weight 71kg	Date of admission : 01/05/20XX

ONCE ONLY AND PRE-MEDICATION DRUGS

Date	Name of drug	Dose	Route	Time to be given	Signature	Given Date	Time	Initials	Pharm
02/05/20XX	TEMAZEPAM	20mg	Oral	07.00	GAMann				

AS REQUIRED AND POST OPERATIVE DRUGS

DRUG APPROVED NAME TRAMADOL	Dose 50mg	Route O	Dose	Date	Time	Dose	Given	Dose	Date	Time	Dose	Given
			1					8				
Frequency QDS	Indication PAIN	Date 02/05/20XX	Pharm	2					9			
				3				10				
Number of doses 6	Detailed directions			4				11				
	Review pain chart			5				12				
Prescriber's signature GAMann				6				13				
				7				14				

REGULAR DRUGS

			Date →							
			Time	Dose						
DRUG APPROVED NAME PHENYTOIN	Route Oral	Frequency Daily	0700							
Prescriber's signature GAMann	Bleep 2664	Pharm	1000							
			1200							
Detailed directions Nocté	Date written 02/05/20XX		1400							
			1700							
	Date cancelled		2200	300mg						
DRUG APPROVED NAME AMOXICILLIN	Route Oral	Frequency QDS	0700	500mg						
Prescriber's signature GAMann	Bleep 2664	Pharm	1000							
			1200	500mg						
Detailed directions	Date written 02/05/20XX		1400							
			1700	500mg						
	Date cancelled		2200	500mg						

Good practice point

Each drug has an approved name (which is universal) but many also have a manufacturer's (brand or trade) name that is specific to each brand. Drugs supplied as 'generics' only have an approved name. Although packaged differently, the drugs contain the same active ingredients. It is good practice to only use the approved 'generic' name (which is usually written in lower-case lettering).

Some labels or *names* of substances may include numbers or percentages as part of the labelling (e.g. 0.9% normal saline or 5% dextrose), and this can be confusing. So it is important you understand which numbers relate to the name of the substance and which are relevant in deciding the strength or dosage. Labels should also include an expiry date for the contents, which you need to check to ensure you do not use expired medicines.

Common sense and estimation

The golden rule of any calculation you make is to have an idea of what a sensible answer should be, before you proceed with the calculation. This becomes much easier with experience, but you will soon develop 'common-sense', or 'number-sense', knowledge if you are reflective in your own practice.

As well as 'common-sense (or number-sense) knowing', you need to make a habit of estimating, especially if the calculation involves decimals or several stages, or if you are using a hand-held calculator. An estimate should be based on the recommended dose range in the formulary used locally (such as the BNF); this is particularly important if you are working with an unfamiliar substance.

In the case of medication calculations and for patient safety, you are just as accountable as the prescriber, and it is not safe to assume that the prescription is automatically correct. Administering an erroneous prescription is committing a medication error, just as much as writing an erroneous prescription.

Methods for calculating medication dosage

Many calculations required in nursing and midwifery will be very straight-forward, and mental arithmetic will be all you need. There are several ways of calculating medication dosages using mental arithmetic and you may feel more comfortable using one over another.

Unit dose

The most straightforward calculations are at unit dose level. In other words, the prescribed dose is the same as the dose (or strength) of the dispensed medicine. Look at the following example of a prescription for an antibiotic:

Date	Name of drug	Dose	Route	Frequency
10/02/20XX	TETRACYCLINE	250 mg	oral	6 hrly

The label on the bottle looks like this:

> Tetracycline Tabs
> 250 mg

Having checked that the prescription is in the same units (mg) as the dispensed drug, we can see immediately that we need 1 tablet to give the prescribed dose of 250 mg. So, we do not need to do a calculation. This is termed a *unit dose*.

Multiple-unit dose

Calculations are really only needed when the prescription is at sub-unit or multiple-unit level; that is, when the prescribed amount is less than the dispensed preparation, or more than the dispensed unit. Let's look at what that really means.

Date	Name of drug	Dose	Route	Frequency
10/02/20XX	TETRACYCLINE	500 mg	oral	b.d. (twice a day)

The label on the bottle reads:

> Tetracycline Tabs
> 250 mg

Here, the prescribed dose is twice the amount contained in one tablet. Common sense tells us that we will need to give 2 tablets, but what if the calculation is not so straightforward? Here's an example.

Worked example 6.1: multiple-unit dose

A patient is prescribed an oral drug to treat an allergic reaction.

Date	Name of drug	Dose	Route	Frequency
10/02/20XX	PREDNISOLONE	25 mg	oral	daily

This would normally be given as a unit dose using one 25 mg strength tablet. In this scenario, the only tablets available have the dose given on the label opposite. How many tablets do we need to give?

Prednisolone
Tabs 10 mg

- *Step 1 – Extract* the required information from the *prescription*:
  We need to administer 25 mg per dose.
- *Step 2 – Check* the formulation and dose on the *product label*:
  The medicine is in tablet form with each tablet containing 10 mg.
  Check: Is the stock medicine in the same units as the prescribed dose?

Yes, both stock and prescription are in milligrams.

- *Step 3 – Estimate*: Do you need more or less than the stock dosage?
  As 25 is larger than 10, we will need more than 1 tablet (10 mg) and indeed more than 2 tablets (20 mg), but less than 3 (30 mg).
- *Step 4 – Calculate* the dose:

Method 1. Look for relationships between the numbers involved. You might note immediately that 25 is $2\frac{1}{2}$ times 10 and that you will need to give $2\frac{1}{2}$ a tablets.

Or:

Method 2. You could reason that if one tablet contains 10 mg, then 2 tablets will contain 20 mg and $\frac{1}{2}$ a tablet will contain 5 mg. Thus, $2\frac{1}{2}$ tablets will provide the required amount of 25 mg.

Or, if you prefer another way (using a formula) to calculate the dose:

Method 3. If you know what quantity contains 1 mg of the drug, then you can multiply it by 25 to find how much you need to give to achieve the prescribed dose. Thus, if 10 mg is contained in 1 tablet, make this into an equation:

10 mg = 1 tablet

To find how much tablet contains 1 mg of drug, divide both sides of the equation by 10:

$1 \text{ mg} = \frac{1}{10}$ of a tablet

Since the prescribed dose is 25 mg, multiply both sides by 25:

$$25 \text{ mg} = \frac{1}{10} \times \frac{25}{1}$$
$$= \frac{25}{10}$$
$$= 2.5 \text{ tablets} \left(2\frac{1}{2}\right).$$

Method 3 may seem overly complicated for this straightforward calculation, but using this step-wise approach may be useful when tackling more difficult calculations.

Irrespective of the method you use, *check* that your answer is around the estimated amount and is a sensible amount to be given by the prescribed route. In this case, we estimated that we needed more than 2 tablets but less than 3, and so our answer of $2\frac{1}{2}$ tablets is reasonable.

Finally, read the 'good practice point' below. Should we be using half a tablet?

 Good practice point

Breaking tablets in half is not considered good practice and neither is breaking tablets to pour powder out. One of the reasons not to break tablets is that some tablets have coatings designed to protect the stomach from the medicine or to prevent the stomach acid from attacking the tablet. These special modifications can be destroyed by crushing or breaking the tablet, and the tablet might have a different effect or may cause side effects if it is altered. It is not possible to tell if a tablet or capsule has a special modifications or coatings just by looking at it.

Sometimes a liquid preparation may be available, which will provide a more reliable measure of the drug. Under no circumstances should you attempt to break enteric-coated (e/c) tablets.

 Good practice point

Sometimes a prescription may read slightly differently from the tablet's label. For example, the prescription may be for 'thiamine' whereas the tablet package is labelled 'Thiamine hydrochloride'. The additional part of the packaging label (i.e. 'hydrochloride') indicates how the active drug is prepared and should not alter the active ingredient. If in doubt, check with the prescriber or refer to a reputable formulary (such as the current BNF) for confirmation that you have the correct preparation.

Sub-unit dose

The dose for a child or an older adult is often less than the unit dose. For example, we may need to administer a dose of Oxycodone Hydrochloride that is under 10 mg, but the stock solution we have contains 10 mg in 5 mL. We would need to work out what volume in mL to administer. We can use the same methods to calculate a sub-unit dose as we did for multiple-unit doses, following steps 1 to 4 shown in **worked example 6.1.** See Chapter 7 for more detail on liquid medication calculations.

Using a formula

As you can see, medication dosage calculations take the form of an equation, where one side equals the other. As demonstrated with the three different methods above, there is no single right way to calculate drug dosages, but there *is* one *formula*, in the form of an equation that always works.

For many sub-unit and multi-unit dosages (with the same units), there is a fairly simple formula that can be applied to work out doses for administration.

$$\frac{\text{what you need}}{\text{what you have}} = \text{dose (in tablets)}$$

This formula will also be revisited and added to in Chapter 7.

Key calculation steps for tablets and capsules

The following complete checklist is one that you should become familiar with, and confident about using, to carry out all basic medication dosage calculations:

- *Step 1 – Extract* the required information from the prescription.
- *Step 2 – Check* the formulation and dose on the *product label*.
  Check that the drug is available in the same units as the prescription.
- *Step 3 – Estimate*: Do you need more or less than the stock dosage?
- *Step 4 – Calculate* using your chosen method.

$$\frac{\text{what you need}}{\text{what you have}} = \text{dose (in tablets)}$$

That is, if a 50 mg dose is needed and you have 25 mg tablets, this would look like:

$\frac{50}{25}$ = 2, so 2 tablets are required.

Alternatively this formula may be written as:

$$\text{number required} = \frac{\text{amount prescribed}}{\text{amount available (in each tablet or capsule)}}$$

- *Step 5 – Check this answer* against the approximation from Step 3 and check that it is a sensible format and amount to be given by the route prescribed.

You will see that many of the dosage calculations involve similar numbers. This is because medications are usually both prescribed and prepared in round numbers, which are easier to calculate. Part of the 'common sense' element to drug calculation is recognizing these numbers and the relationships between them, something that will become easier with regular practice.

Chapter summary

This chapter has discussed calculations and drug administration with tablets and capsules, but not all medication is in a solid format. The following chapters explore calculations related to liquid medicines and doses based on body weight.

Medications safety: administering liquid medications and prescriptions based on weight

This chapter covers:

- Liquid medications
- Additional checks when administering medicines for children and older adults
- Considering a patient's weight when administering drugs

Liquid medications

We have already looked at different ways of how to calculate straightforward prescriptions for tablets and capsules. However, many drugs used for children are prepared as liquids. This makes them easier to give in a range of doses, as would be required for children of different ages and sizes. The same methods that we used for calculating tablets and capsules can be applied to calculate liquid medicines. But how does the method that we reported in the previous chapter work for liquids? Here is an example.

Worked example 7.1: liquid medication (i)

A toddler is prescribed the antibiotic flucloxacillin for an ear infection.

Date	Name of drug	Dose	Route	Frequency
10/02/20XX	FLUCLOXACILLIN	125 mg	oral	4 × daily

The label on the bottle reads:

> Flucloxacillin
> syrup 125 mg
> in 5 mL

This drug is available in syrup form, 125 mg in 5 mL. This is the unit dose, the liquid equivalent of 1 tablet. How much should you administer?

- *Step 1 – Extract* the required information from the prescription.
- *Step 2 – Check* the formulation and dose on the *product label.*
  Check that the drug is available in the same units as the prescription.
- *Step 3 – Estimate*: Do you need more or less than the stock dosage?
- *Step 4 – Calculate using your chosen method.*

$$\frac{\text{what you want}}{\text{what you have}} = \text{dose}$$

- *Step 5 – Check this answer* against the approximation from Step 3 and check that it is a sensible format and amount to be given by the route prescribed.

The answer is of course 5 mL.

But what if the prescription is for a different amount?

Date	Name of drug	Dose	Route	Frequency
10/02/20XX	FLUCLOXACILLIN	250 mg	oral	4 × daily

This drug is available in syrup form, 125 mg in 5 mL. How much should you give?

- *Steps 1 and 2* – Check the information from the prescription and the formulation and dose on the *product label.*
- *Step 3 – Estimate*: Do you need more or less than the stock dosage?
  The prescribed dose of 250 mg is more than the unit dose on the bottle and so we will need to administer more than 5 mL.
- *Step 4 – Calculate using your chosen method.* We will give examples based on the three methods described in Chapter 6.

Method 1. You can probably see that 250 is 2 × 125 and so a dose of 10 mL (twice the 'unit' 5 mL) is required.

Method 2. If 5 mL contains 125 mg, then we need twice as much (10 mL) to get 250 mg.

Method 3. If 125 mg = 5 mL, then

$$1 \text{ mg} = \frac{5}{125} \text{ mL}$$

$$250 \text{ mg} = \frac{5}{125} \times 250 \text{ mL}$$

$$250 \text{ mg} = \frac{1250}{125} \text{ mL}$$

$$250 \text{ mg} = 10 \text{ mL}.$$

Would using the formula give this answer? Applying the formula

$$\frac{\text{what you need}}{\text{what you have}} = \text{dose},$$

substitute the known values to get your answer:

$$\frac{\text{what you need}}{\text{what you have}} = \frac{250}{125}$$

Simplify the fraction by dividing both top and bottom by 25:

$$\frac{\cancel{250}^{\,10}}{\cancel{125}_{\,5}}$$

Or by 5 several times if you prefer:

$$\frac{\cancel{250}^{\,\cancel{50}^{10}}}{\cancel{125}_{\,\cancel{25}_{5}}} \text{ gives } \frac{10}{5} = 2$$

So, from the formula, the answer is 2.

- *Step 5 – Check this answer* against the approximation from Step 3 and check that it is a sensible format and amount to be given by the route prescribed. We estimated that the dose would be more than 5 mL and so 2 mL cannot be right. So, from the formula, the answer must be two '*of what*'.

Remember that each 125 mg dose of drug that we have *is contained in 5 mL of liquid* and so the answer is two portions of 5 mL, so the dose required is a total of 10 mL. Thus, to get a sensible answer, we have to multiply the formula by the measure (or volume) that the available drug is supplied in.

In the previous chapter we were working with tablets and capsules, where the unit dose was always *one* tablet or capsule, so we were effectively multiplying by 1.

Let's add this to the formula to make it work for every type of prescription which can be remembered as 'NHS1':

$$\text{Dose} = \frac{\text{what you Need}}{\text{what you Have}} \times \frac{\text{Stock volume}}{1} = \text{dose in mL}$$

Remember that we can put a 1 in the denominator for the stock dose. This does not change the value of the stock number, because any number divided by 1 does not itself change, e.g. $4 \div 1 = 4$. Adding the 1 will help to maintain accuracy in solving the calculation, and makes the sum look more like a balanced equation.

Check by substituting the values we have above:

$$\text{Dose} = \frac{250}{125} \times \frac{5}{1}$$

Cancel down to simplify, for example, we can divide both top and bottom by 25 to get $\frac{10}{5} \times \frac{5}{1}$.

We can simplify further, by cancelling the 5s top and bottom to leave $\frac{10}{1} = 10$. So, the dose required is 10 mL.

Check: Is this a sensible answer close to our estimate? Yes.

Let's try using the revised formula again, this time for a sub-unit dose.

Worked example 7.2: liquid medication (II)

Date	Name of drug	Dose	Route	Frequency
10/02/20XX	IBUPROFEN	50 mg	oral	3 × daily

The label on the bottle reads:

> Ibuprofen
> Oral Suspension
> 100 mg in 5 mL

- *Step 1 – Extract* the required information from the prescription.
- *Step 2 – Check* the formulation and dose on the *product label*.
  Check that the drug is available in the same units as the prescription.
- *Step 3 – Estimate*: Do you need more or less than the stock dosage?
  The prescribed dose of 50 mg is less than the unit dose on the bottle and so we will need less than 5 mL.
- *Step 4 – Calculate by applying the revised formula.*

$$\text{Dose} = \frac{\text{what you Need}}{\text{what you Have}} \times \frac{\text{Stock volume}}{1} = \text{dose in mL}$$

Substitute the known quantities:

$$\text{Dose} = \frac{50}{100} \times \frac{5}{1} \text{ mL}$$

Cancel down by dividing top and bottom by 10 to get:

$$\frac{5}{10} \times \frac{5}{1} \, \text{mL}$$

Then multiply across both the top line and the bottom line:

$$= \frac{25}{10} \, \text{mL}$$

$$= 2\frac{5}{10} \, \text{mL and simplified this is 2.5 mL.}$$

- *Step 5 – Check this answer* against the approximation from Step 3 and check that it is a sensible format and amount to be given by the route prescribed.

Is it sensible? Yes.

Good practice point

When preparing liquid medicines, especially for children, the volumes may be quite small. In this situation, it is recommended that you measure the liquid medicine using a suitable syringe, rather than the conventional medicine pot.

Additional check before dispensing medications to children or older adults

Normal adult doses of medications are unsuitable for administering to children in the majority of cases. Such doses may also be unsuitable for frail, immune-compromised or older adults. There is an additional check we can do against the prescription, which is useful in adult nursing and strongly recommended in children's nursing or if nursing older adults. This check is absolutely essential for prescribers, but also safeguards the person administering the medication from dosage errors made in the prescription.

Good practice point

Use the recommended dose range and/or recommended maximum dose given in the local formulary to check that the prescribed amount is sensible, remembering to take into account the size of the patient, route prescribed, and frequency of the dose.

Worked example 7.3: additional check when administering for older adults

Below is an extract from the prescription chart of an older adult patient who is newly diagnosed with Alzheimer's disease.

Date	Name of drug	Dose	Route	Frequency
10/02/20XX	RIVASTIGMINE	1.5 mg	oral (by syringe)	twice daily (b.d.)

- *Step 1 – Extract* the required information from the prescription.

  Drug name rivastigmine (used to treat mild dementia in Alzheimer's disease).
- *Step 2 – Check* the formulation and dose on the *product label.*

  Check that the drug is available in the same units as the prescription.

  Liquid format to be given orally.

  Dose 1.5 mg.

  Check the prescription, especially if unfamiliar with the drug or dealing with children or older adults.

The British National Formulary (BNF) suggests an initial dose of 1.5 mg rivastigmine twice daily, increasing to the usual range of 3–6 mg twice daily and maximum 6 mg twice daily. Does this prescription fall within the recommended range?

Yes, the prescribed dose of 1.5 mg twice a day is in line with the recommended dose.

Check that the drug is available in the same units as the prescription:

The label on the bottle in stock reads:

> Rivastigmine
> Oral Solution
> 2 mg per mL

Having identified that the prescription is in the right range for our patient, and that we have the right drug for the correct route of administration, we can focus on the information that is directly relevant to the calculation – the prescribed dose and the strength of the stock preparation.

- *Step 3 – Estimate*: Do you need more or less than the stock dosage?

  The prescribed amount of 1.5 mg is less than 2 mg.

  As the stock solution is 2 mg in 1 mL, we need less than 1 mL.

- *Step 4 – Calculate using your chosen method.*

  Method 1. Look for relationships between the numbers involved.
  You may recognize that 1.5 is $\frac{3}{4}$ of 2.

  So, if there are 2 mg in 1 mL, there will be 1.5 mg in $\frac{3}{4}$ of 1 mL.
  Required amount = 0.75 mL.

  Method 2. Logic tells you that if there is 2 mg in 1 mL, then there will be 1 mg
  in $\frac{1}{2}$ mL and 0.5 mg in half of that (i.e. $\frac{1}{4}$ mL).
  So you will need $\frac{1}{2} + \frac{1}{4}$ mL = $\frac{3}{4}$ mL or 0.75 mL.

  Method 3. If you know what quantity contains 1 mg of the drug, then you
  can multiply it by 1.5 to calculate the volume containing 1.5 mg.
  The label 2 mg per mL tells us that 1 mg is in $\frac{1}{2}$ mL or 0.5 mL.

  If 1 mg = 0.5 mL, then 1.5 mg = 0.5 × 1.5 = 0.75.
  Required amount is = 0.75 mL.

  Method 4. Apply the formula:

  $$\text{Dose} = \frac{\text{what you need}}{\text{what you have}} \times \frac{\text{stock volume}}{1}$$

  Substitute known values:

  $$\text{Dose} = \frac{1.5}{2} \times \frac{1}{1} \text{mL}$$

  Remove the decimal by multiplying top and bottom by 10:

  $$= \frac{15}{20} \times 1 \text{mL}$$

  Cancel down by dividing top and bottom by 5:

  $$= \frac{3}{4} \text{ mL or 0.75 mL}$$

- *Step 5 – Check this answer* against the approximation from Step 3.

Is it a sensible format and amount to be given by the prescribed route? Yes.

Prescriptions based on weight

In neonatal and children's nursing, and when prescribing cytotoxic drugs for
cancer, the weight of the patient is of paramount importance and doses may
differ widely due to the patient's weight. Checking the prescription is particularly important when medication is prescribed in relation to a patient's weight.
There is an additional calculation to be made when doing this.

Worked example 7.4: prescription based on weight

A 4-year-old child, weighing 25.5 kg, is to have the antibiotic amoxicillin orally, three times a day, for treatment of otitis media (a middle ear infection).

Date	Name of drug	Dose	Route	Frequency
10/02/20XX	AMOXICILLIN	250 mg	oral	t.d.s.

Remember there is an *additional stage* for safety in medication calculations, particularly relevant to children or dose by weight, and so the calculation process is as follows:

- *Step 1 – Extract* the required information from the prescription.
- *Step 2 – Check* the formulation and dose on the *product label.*
  Check the prescription, especially if unfamiliar with the drug or dealing with children or older adults.
  Check that the drug is available in the same units as the prescription.

The label on the bottle reads:

> Amoxicillin
> 125 mg/1.25 mL Oral
> Sugar-free Suspension

- *Step 3 – Estimate*: Do you need more or less than the stock dosage?
- *Step 4 – Calculate using your chosen method.*
- *Step 5 – Check this answer* against the approximation from Step 3 and check that it is a sensible format and amount to be given by the route prescribed.

So let's work this through.

- *Step 1 – Extract* the required information from the prescription.
  The child is prescribed 250 mg amoxicillin orally three times a day.
- *Step 2 – Check* the formulation and dose on the *product label.*
  Check the prescription, especially if unfamiliar with the drug or dealing with children or older adults.
  Check that the drug is available in the same units as the prescription.

The British National Formulary (BNF) states that oral amoxicillin should be prescribed to children aged 1 to 4 years with otitis media at a dose of 250 mg three times daily and increase if necessary up to 30 milligrams per kilogram (mg/kg) three times daily, to be given in three divided doses (maximum 1 g daily).

This information gives us a number of check points:

- type of infection
- a suggested dose and a dose per weight of the child
- the maximum recommended dose.

So is the prescription above within the recommended range for our patient? We need to calculate a number of things:

(**a**) Correct daily dose and whether it is within the recommended maximum.
(**b**) Correct divided dose.
(**c**) Amount of drug to administer each time, based on the available preparation.

Taking these in turn:

(**a**) We need to find the correct daily dose for a child of this weight.
The child weighs 25.5 kg.
Recommended dose is 250 mg three times a day, which is 750 mg, or 30 mg per kg. If we work out the per kg amount, this tells us that the *daily* dose should be:
$30 \times 25.5 = 765$ mg.
Is this within the recommended daily maximum? Yes, 1 g is the recommended daily maximum.
Because 1 g = 1000 mg and so the amount calculated (765 mg) is well within the recommended maximum.
(**b**) To continue with this second example, the daily dose now needs to be divided into three equal doses.
$765 \div 3 = 255$ mg, and so each dose should be 255 mg.
(**c**) It would not be sensible to prescribe this exact amount, as it would result in a volume of 2.55 mL, which is difficult to measure accurately. It is therefore sensible to prescribe a more easily calculated and measured volume such as 250 mg, which matches the prescription.

We can now move on to the next stage:

Check that the drug is available in the same units as the prescription.

Amoxicillin is available as:

> Amoxicillin
> 125 mg/1.25 mL Oral
> Sugar-free Suspension

This is in the same units as the prescription (milligrams).

- *Step 3 – Estimate* an approximate answer: Do you need more or less than the stock dosage?
As the prescription is for 250 mg, we will need more than the unit dose on the bottle. By approximating the 1.25 to 1, we can see that we will need at least 2 mL.
- *Step 4 – Calculate using your chosen method.*

$$\text{Dose} = \frac{\text{what you need}}{\text{what you have}} \times \frac{\text{stock volume}}{1} = \text{dose in mL}$$

which gives us $\dfrac{250}{125} \times \dfrac{1.25}{1} = \text{dose in mL}$

This is a mixture of fractions and decimals and so we need to simplify the fraction. We can do this by cancelling down by dividing the top and bottom by 125, or dividing in stages by 5 or 25, to get: $2 \times 1.25 = 2.5$ mL.

- *Step 5* – Finally, we should check the answer.

Key calculation steps for liquids and prescriptions based on patient's weight

The following steps have been modified – from the method outlined in Chapter 6 – to assist with calculations for liquids and weight-based prescriptions.

- *Step 1* – *Extract* the required information from the prescription.
- *Step 2* – *Check* the formulation and dose on the *product label*.
  Check the prescription, especially if unfamiliar with the drug or dealing with children or older adults.
  Check that the drug is available in the same units as the prescription.
- *Step 3* – *Estimate* an approximate answer: Do you need more or less than the stock dosage?
- *Step 4* – *Calculate* using your chosen method.

$$\text{Dose} = \frac{\text{what you need}}{\text{what you have}} \times \frac{\text{stock volume}}{1} = \text{dose in mL}$$

Alternatively this formula may be written as:

$$\text{Volume required} = \frac{\text{strength prescribed}}{\text{strength available}} \times \frac{\text{volume of stock}}{1}$$

- *Step 5* – *Check this answer* against the approximation from Step 3 and check that it is a sensible format and amount to be administered by the route prescribed.

Chapter summary

This chapter has covered prescriptions in which a patient's weight must be considered, as is often required for paediatric patients. In some cases it is more accurate to calculate a therapeutic dose using the body's surface area as a guide, although this is a less commonly used format and so will be covered in Chapter 10.

8 | Medications safety: injections, IV fluids, and drip rates

> This chapter covers:
>
> - Medication by injection
> - Appropriate volumes and routes of administration for injection (subcutaneous, intramuscular, intravenous, into airway, epidural)
> - IV therapy – drip rates for blood and clear fluids using manual sets and volumetric pumps
> - Syringe drivers

Injections

Medication is given by injection for a number of reasons. It may be because the preparation is not suitable for enteral use (via the gastro-intestinal tract), the patient may be unable to take the medicine by mouth, or it may be that more rapid absorption is required. Healthcare practitioners may be required to give, or assist with the giving of, injections by the following routes:

- *intramuscular* – into the muscle, usually outer arm, thigh or buttocks;
- *subcutaneous* – into subcutaneous tissue, usually abdomen, outer arm or thigh;
- *intradermal* – into the dermis of the skin, usually inner arm, upper back or upper chest;
- *intravenous* – directly into a vein;
- *epidural* – into the epidural space, via the back;
- *intrathecal* – into the cerebrospinal fluid (CSF), via the back;
- *via airway* – inhaled into bronchi.

The route of administration of the injection will influence the volume of drug that can be administered. Injections directly into the blood stream (intravenous) can be of a larger volume than an intramuscular or subcutaneous injection. For example, when anaesthetic is injected into the epidural space, it is intended to give anaesthesia below the level of injection; however, if too much anaesthetic is administered, it will disperse upwards and may cause total paralysis and death. Therefore, the nurse has to employ common sense when preparing and/or checking any drug for injection and to recognize what is a sensible amount to give via that particular route. Large amounts of medicine injected into muscle or subcutaneously can be very painful.

 Good practice point

It is the responsibility of all registered healthcare professionals to ensure they are dealing with medication as stipulated in the relevant guidelines for their profession. This means you may need to be supervised in administering medication. For patient safety, and your own professional accountability, it is important to always be aware of the current rules guiding practice in your profession.

This is an additional check to be made when calculating the dosage of injections (see Table 8.1). Otherwise, the method for calculating dosage of drugs for injection is the same as calculating liquid drug dosages to be administered orally.

Table 8.1 Types of injections

Route of injection	Typical volume (in adults)	Example
Intramuscular (IM)	1–3 mL	Analgesics, anti-emetics, sedatives, immunizations
Subcutaneous (SC)	0.5–1 mL	Heparin and insulin
Intradermal (ID)	Up to 0.5 mL	Sensitivity tests, local anaesthetics
Intravenous (IV)	Variable 0–500 mL	Antibiotics, analgesia
Epidural	Up to 10 mL (block to groin) 15–20 mL (block to upper abdomen)	Local anaesthetics/ analgesia, opiates
Intrathecal (spinal, only for specialist administration)	2–4 mL	Local anaesthetic/analgesia
Via airway	1–2 puffs/1–5 mL via a nebuliser	Topical bronchodilators

As with oral medicines, you should carry out injection dosage calculations in the following stages:

- *Step 1 – Extract* the required information from the prescription.
- *Step 2 – Check* the formulation and dose on the *product label*.

  Check the prescription, especially if unfamiliar with the drug or dealing with children or older adults.

  Check that the drug is available in the same units as the prescription.
- *Step 3 – Estimate* an approximate answer: Do you need more or less than the stock dosage?
- *Step 4 – Calculate using your chosen method.*

$$\text{Volume required} = \frac{\text{strength prescribed}}{\text{strength available}} \times \frac{\text{volume of stock}}{1}$$

- *Step 5 – Check this answer* against the approximation from Step 3 and check that it is a sensible format and amount to be administered by the route prescribed.

Worked example 8.1: Injections

A frail older adult patient is prescribed intramuscular codeine phosphate for relief of pain.

Date	Name of drug	Dose	Route	Frequency
10/02/20XX	CODEINE PHOSPHATE	45 mg	IM	4 times a day

Codeine Phosphate is available as:

Codeine Phosphate
60 mg/mL

- *Step 1 – Extract* the required information from the prescription.

  We need 45 mg of codeine phosphate.
- *Step 2 – Check* the formulation and dose on the *product label*.

  Check the prescription, especially if unfamiliar with the drug or dealing with children or older adults.

The BNF information on codeine phosphate advises 30–60 mg 4 hourly as necessary, to a maximum of 240 mg daily. The prescribed amount of 45 mg four times a day would result in a total of 4 × 45 mg (180 mg) over 24 hours, which is within the daily maximum.

Check that the drug is available in the same units as the prescription.

Yes, the prescription is in mg and so is the dispensed product.

- *Step 3 – Estimate* an approximate answer: Do you need more or less than the stock dosage?

  The required amount is less than the unit dose, but more than half of it and so we need an amount between 0.5 and 1 mL.

- *Step 4 – Calculate using your chosen method.*

  The first two methods (described in previous chapters) are not as easy for this particular dose because there is no obvious relationship between the prescribed dose and the available preparation. So here we will use method 3.

Method 3. If you know the volume of the liquid that contains 1 mg of the drug, then multiply it by 45, to calculate the volume containing 45 mg:

60 mg = 1 mL

By dividing both sides of the equation by 60:

$$1 \text{ mg} = \frac{1}{60} \text{ mL.}$$

Thus $45 \text{ mg} = 45 \times \frac{1}{60} \text{ mL.}$

Cancel down by dividing top and bottom by 15:

$$= \frac{3}{4} \text{ mL} = 0.75 \text{ mL.}$$

Formula: $\dfrac{\text{what you need}}{\text{what you have}} \times \dfrac{\text{stock volume}}{1} = \text{dose.}$

Substitute from the prescription to get:

$$\frac{45}{60} \times \frac{1}{1} = \frac{45}{60} = \frac{3}{4} \text{ mL} = 0.75 \text{ mL}$$

- *Step 5 – Check this answer* against the approximation from Step 3 and check that it is a sensible format and amount to be given by the route prescribed.

> ✒ **Good practice point**
>
> For optimum accuracy, always use a syringe size as near as possible to the volume of the injection. To draw up 0.75 mL, use a 1 mL syringe if possible (Figure 8.1).

Figure 8.1 A 1 mL syringe filled to 0.75 mL

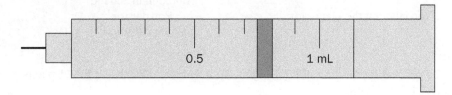

0.5   1 mL

Displacement in reconstituted powders

Some injectable drugs are stored as a powder and have to be reconstituted (restored) to a liquid before being given. This liquid is called the *diluent*, or sometimes, *dilutent*.

Common diluents are normal saline (0.9% sodium chloride) and 'Water for Injection' (a specially prepared form of distilled water, used for parenteral administration). Both the diluent and the powder containing the active ingredient of the preparation must be sterile.

 Good practice point

Dissolving a powder in a volume of liquid may increase the volume of the liquid as the powder displaces the diluent. It is important to remember this when reconstituting powdered drugs.

A prescription for 250 mg amoxicillin, when prepared for intramuscular injection, may be reconstituted from powder (250 mg) by adding 1.5 mL of Water for Injection (this is the diluent). The result of this reconstitution is a prepared medication with a volume of 1.7 mL. This volume difference (in this example it is 0.2 mL) does not matter, except when the reconstituted medicine is not being given in its entirety (when only part of the medicine is required). In this case, it is important to allow for the displacement when calculating the final volume to give. The reconstituted volume may be given in the product literature, or a displacement value may be quoted. If working with the displacement value, it must be added to the amount of diluent, to give the final volume.

Worked example 8.2: reconstitution of powdered drug

Amoxicillin prescribed for a 10 kg child.

Date	Name of drug	Dose	Route	Frequency
10/02/20XX	AMOXICILLIN	125 mg	IM	6 hrly

The label on the vial reads:

> Amoxicillin 250 mg
> Powder for
> Reconstitution

The product literature will inform you of the correct diluent and the displacement value, if any.

The product information preparation instructions for amoxicillin are:

Amoxicillin 250 mg Intramuscular injection – add *1.5 mL of Water for Injection.* Shake vigorously. Final volume is *1.7 mL.*

Water for Injection 2 mL ⊏⊐

- *Extract* the required information:

    In this case, it is not only the prescription sheet and the labels that are providing information but also the product literature and/or the local pharmacy guidelines.
- *Check the prescription.* The BNF recommendation is as follows:

    Intramuscular amoxicillin, CHILD, 50–100 mg/kg daily in divided doses.

    What is the recommended daily dose for a child of 10 kg?
    According to this information, it is between 10 × 50 mg and 10 × 100 mg.
    Or 500–1000 mg over 24 hours.
    The patient has been prescribed 125 mg, given 6 hourly.
    This gives a total amount over 24 hours of 4 × 125 mg = 500 mg. This is within the recommended range.
- *Check* that the drug is available in the same units as the prescription.

    Yes, both prescription and preparation are in milligrams.
- *Estimate* an approximate answer:

    By adding 1.5 mL of water to the vial we will have reconstituted 250 mg of amoxicillin in 1.7 mL.
    We need 125 mg and so we are going to need half the reconstituted vial.
- *Calculate using your chosen method:*

$$\frac{\text{what you need}}{\text{what you have}} \times \frac{\text{stock volume}}{1} = \text{dose in mL.}$$

Substitute the known values to get your answer:

$$\frac{\cancel{125}^{1}}{\cancel{250}_{2}} \times \frac{1.7}{1} = \frac{1.7}{2}$$
$$= 0.85 \text{ mL}$$

- *Check this answer* against your approximation and check that it is a sensible format and amount to be given by the route prescribed.

Intravenous fluids and calculating a drip rate

Intravenous (IV) fluids are given to patients for a number of reasons. If patients are unable to ingest sufficient fluid orally because of their condition, they are likely to have all or some of the daily requirement of fluid via an intravenous infusion, often referred to as a 'drip'. Some other reasons for having IV fluids are to receive a blood transfusion, other blood products such as platelets or plasma, potent drugs such as cytotoxic therapy, or intravenous feeding.

The flow rate is generally defined as the 'number of millilitres of fluid to be administered over 1 hour' (mL/hr) (although it can also refer to the number of millilitres to be delivered over a minute).

Normally, the flow of an infusion is regulated automatically by an electronic infusion device, such as a volumetric infusion pump. These automatic devices generally require programming, and a calculation may be required to convert the prescribed dose and time into the infusion rate – the number of drops per minute (in mL/hr). The formula below can be used to programme and check electronic infusion devices.

$$\text{Rate (mL/hr)} = \frac{\text{Volume (mL)}}{\text{Time (hrs)}}$$

Check Appendix D for one way to remember this formula.

A prescription for intravenous fluids might look something like this:

Fluid	Volume	Duration	Start time/date
Dextrose 5%	1 litre	6 hours	13.00 21/01/20XX

To be able to set up this infusion correctly, you need to know about the equipment available and what it does.

The easiest equipment to use is a volumetric infusion pump, most of which can be used to set the volume to be infused in millilitres and the rate per hour giving a rate of millilitres per hour (mL/hr). This still requires a calculation by the person setting it up to convert the prescribed amount and time into mL/hr.

Worked example 8.3: volumetric infusion pump

To set up the drip rate, you need to enter the correct information into the pump. We follow the same process as that used to calculate prescribed medication doses:

- *Extract* the relevant information from the prescription for IV fluids above.
  The fluid prescribed is 5% dextrose and the rate is 1 litre over 6 hours.
  Is the 5% something that you need to account for in your calculation?

No – in this case, 5% dextrose is just the name of the fluid prescribed.

- *Check* that the drug is available in the same units as the prescription.

  This can be interpreted as: 'Are the units of the prescription the same units as the delivery device (volumetric pump)?'

  No, we have 1 litre of fluid and the pump requires us to enter millilitres. So, we need to convert the prescription to the units used by the pump:

  1 litre = 1000 mL.

  The prescription time is in hours and we have to enter hours on the pump, so that is fine.

- *Estimate* an approximate answer:

  We need to work out how a rate of 1000 mL in 6 hours is converted to mL/hr. The rate of anything depends on what it is and the time taken. For example, the rate of a car is the distance it travels divided by the time taken:

  $$60 \text{ miles in 2 hours} = \frac{60}{2} = 30 \text{ mph.}$$

  The rate of an intravenous infusion is the volume delivered divided by the time taken:

  $$\text{Rate} = \frac{\text{Volume}}{\text{Time}}$$

  $$1000 \text{ mL in 6 hrs} = \frac{1000}{6} \text{ mL/hr}$$

  To approximate, it is easier to divide 1000 by 5, which equals 200.

- *Calculate*:

  $$\frac{\cancel{1000}^{500}}{\cancel{6}_3} = \frac{500}{3} = 166.666 \text{ mL/hr}$$

- *Check* this against the estimated rate.

NB: The pump shown (in Figure 8.2) allows us to enter a decimal point, but with other pumps we may need to round up or down to the nearest whole number.

- *Final check* that you have the correct fluid and the correct volume.

NB: Other checks have to be made before setting up an IV infusion but they do not affect the calculation element and so will not be discussed here.

To set the pump, enter 1000 on the pump control panel (Figure 8.2) as the volume to be infused and the rate as close to the calculated value as the device will accept. Some pumps will only allow whole numbers to be entered and so any decimals in the calculated rate need to be rounded (see Chapter 3 for rounding rules). Pumps used in paediatric units may allow a decimal point to be entered. Usually only one decimal place is used and so you need to correct your calculation to one decimal place. In this example we would enter 166.7.

Figure 8.2 A typical volumetric infusion pump control panel

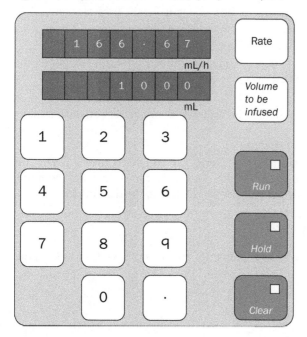

Having set volume and rate, we rely on the electronic pump to deliver the fluid to the patient at the correct rate.

Calculating a manual drip rate

In certain situations, automatic pumps may not be available, and infusions (or fluid replacement therapy) must be administered by a manual infusion under the influence of gravity.

We have to try to set the rate as accurately as possible to start with, by hand. We can set the drip rate manually by adjusting the roller on the tubing of the intravenous giving set (Figure 8.3) and counting the drops as they enter the drip chamber. To do this, we need to know how to calculate the number of drops to be delivered over a period for which it is reasonable to stand there and measure. Hence, to set up a manual infusion accurately, it is sensible to set a drop rate in terms of the number of *drops per minute*.

Calculating the number of drops per minute depends on the volume to be infused in terms of drops – that is, we need to know the size or volume of each drop or how many drips are in a millilitre. We also need to consider the characteristics of the giving set used in the infusion; the size of the drop delivered by every IV giving set should be written on its packaging.

Figure 8.3 An intravenous giving set attached to a bag of fluid

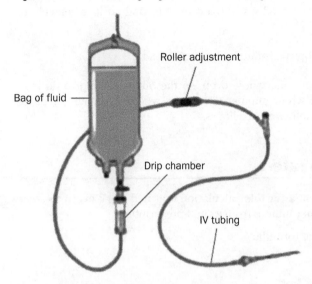

Roller adjustment

Bag of fluid

Drip chamber

IV tubing

Standard giving sets are either macro-drip sets, with a drip factor of 20 drops/mL for clear fluids (or 15 drops/mL for blood – proof that blood is thicker than water!) or micro-drip sets, which deliver a drip rate of 60 drops/mL. Macro-drip sets are used in situations that require infusions of large volumes, while micro-drip sets can be used for children or to administer smaller volumes with more accuracy and are sometimes called 'paediatric giving sets'.

The standard formula for checking manual infusions is as follows:

$$\text{Drip rate (drops/min)} = \frac{\text{drops/mL of the giving set} \times \text{volume}}{\text{number of hours to run} \times 60}$$

Worked example 8.4: manual drip rates

We have already calculated the rate for 1000 mL of clear fluid to be delivered over 6 hours using the volumetric pump and we got 166.67 mL/hr (correct to two decimal places). To calculate the rate of drops per minute, we need to convert the millilitres into drops and the hours into minutes.

First, convert the millilitres into drops. Assuming that the giving set delivers 20 drops to a millilitre, 166.67 mL will be:

166.67 × 20 drops/litre = 3333.4 drops per hour

Next change the hour into minutes. There are 60 minutes in one hour, so divide by 60 to get the rate per minute.

Check that this is sensible. At a set rate, an amount delivered over a minute will be less than an amount delivered over an hour and so it is sensible to divide:

$3333.4 \div 60 = 55.56$ drops per minute

We cannot count less than one whole drop, so the obvious thing to do is to round this to the nearest whole number. Therefore, we need to count 56 drops per minute to get 1 litre delivered in 6 hours.

Formula for drop rate

Can we construct a formula for this calculation that will work every time we need to calculate drops per minute from a fluid prescription?

We already have the basic formula:

$$\text{Rate} = \frac{\text{Volume}}{\text{Time}}$$

but this gave us a rate of millilitres per hour.

To get drops per minute, multiply the volume in millilitres by the number of drops per mL and divided by 60 to get minutes rather than hours:

$$\text{Rate} = \frac{\text{Volume}}{\text{Time}} \times \frac{\text{drops per mL}}{60}$$

Worked example 8.5: manual drip rate using formula

Mrs Noon needs a unit of packed blood cells.

Fluid	Volume	Duration	Giving set drop factor
Packed cells	400 mL	2 hours	15 drops/mL

Use the formula to calculate the rate at which to set the infusion:

$$\text{Rate} = \frac{\text{Volume}}{\text{Time}} \times \frac{\text{drops per mL}}{60}$$

Substitute the known values in the equation to get:

$$\text{Rate} = \frac{400}{2} \times \frac{15}{60} = 50 \text{ drops per minute}$$

Worked example 8.6: drip rate over half an hour

David needs an antibiotic given intravenously over half an hour.

Fluid	Volume	Duration	Giving set drop factor
Vancomycin 500 mg	100 mL	30 mins	20 drops/mL

$$\text{Rate} = \frac{\text{Volume}}{\text{Time}} \times \frac{\text{drops per mL}}{60}$$

Note that the formula allows for conversion of hours to minutes, which is not needed in this case as the time is already given in minutes. So the formula becomes:

$$\text{Rate} = \frac{\text{Volume}}{\text{Time}} \times \text{drops per mL}$$

Substitute known values:

$$\text{Rate} = \frac{100}{30} \times \frac{20}{1} = \frac{2000}{3} = 66.6$$

As this number refers to drops, it needs to be rounded up to 67 drops per minute.

Syringe drivers

A syringe driver or syringe pump is an electronically controlled device that depresses the plunger of a horizontal syringe at a constant set rate. It allows constant delivery of small amounts over a set period of time. Rate of delivery depends on the type of device, and normally the calculation required for the rate is for millilitres per hour. However, some devices are designed to allow the plunger to move a measured distance over time and so deliver the content contained within *millimetres* of syringe length per unit of time, rather than volume. The nurse needs to measure the length of the fluid column in the syringe to set the correct rate. This will of course depend on the size and make of syringe and requires a great deal of care to ensure correct dosages are given.

In neonates and intensive care environments, intravenous medication may be delivered via a syringe driver where delivery needs to be slower than can be controlled by hand or the amount is too much to give as a *bolus*. Special training is recommended for the use of syringe drivers, since their incorrect operation is a frequent cause of drug errors.

In most hospital units, electronic syringe drivers are used, which, with the correct syringe inserted, can be programmed to deliver millilitres per hour. The examples given here will refer to this type of device. Syringe drivers may be used for constant delivery of a drug or for intermittent delivery at specified intervals.

Worked example 8.7: syringe driver rates

An adult prescription for endocarditis, a severe infection of the heart lining, is:

Name of drug	Dose	Route	Frequency
AMOXICILLIN	2 g	IV	6 hourly

- *Extract* the required information from the prescription sheet, the labels and the product literature, and/or the local pharmacy guidelines.

The label on the vial reads:

> Amoxicillin 1 g
> Powder for
> Reconstitution

The label on the ampoule reads:

> Water for Injection 20 mL

The product literature/pharmacy guidelines suggest reconstitution as follows:

Amoxicillin for IV infusion – give over 30 minutes to 1 hour.

Add 20 mL Water for Injection to 1 g powder, final volume 20.8 mL.

- *Check* that the drug is available in the same units as the prescription.
  Both prescription and preparation are in grams.
- *Estimate* an approximate answer:
  By adding 20 mL of water to the vial we will have reconstituted 1 g of amoxicillin. We need 2 g and so we are going to have to use 2 vials and 2 ampoules of water and so it will be approximately 40 mL.
- *Calculate using your chosen method*:
  This one is quite straightforward. By reconstituting as directed, we will get:

  1 g in 20.8 mL, thus

  2 g in 2 × 20.8 mL = 41.6 mL.
- *Check this answer* against the approximation and check that it is a sensible format and amount to be given by the route prescribed.

Now we have to set the syringe driver to deliver the drug at an appropriate rate. This is a case of intermittent delivery (every 6 hours) but over 30 minutes to an hour. As the volume we have calculated is nearly 42 mL, it would be appropriate to set the syringe driver to 42 mL/hour.

Chapter summary

This chapter has covered common calculations related to injections, IV fluids, and drip rates. The next chapter will look at the types of calculations you may encounter when monitoring patients' fluid balance.

Part **3**

Specialized calculation skills

q Fluid balance calculations

This chapter covers:

- General fluid balance
- Special cases – irrigation and dialysis
- Fluid balance in children

Calculations related to fluid balance are usually straightforward, as they require only addition and subtraction. However, the healthcare practitioner will also need to have an understanding of measurements associated with weight, volume, and time. In children's nursing, and when nursing neonates, the calculations can become more complicated.

The chapter will begin by looking at fluid balance calculations used in adult nursing and then progress to the more difficult calculations required for specialist situations.

A healthy body maintains a dynamic balance between fluid and electrolyte intake and loss. A 24-hour period (1 day) is considered as a suitable period over which a balance should be maintained. In other words, the amount of fluid taken in over 24 hours should equal the amount being lost through all routes. Many conditions affect an individual's ability to maintain this balance, both physical and psychological, and, as a healthcare practitioner, you are almost certain to come across patients/clients in whom the balance is upset. Maintaining fluid balance is therefore a common and important component of nursing duties.

Minimal fluid requirements vary from person to person depending on their size and level of activity. Patients in hospital may have specific needs and so their requirements can differ from those published. For example, if a patient is already dehydrated, he or she will need more fluid than the standard stated requirement and the aim will be to end up in a positive balance at the end of the day. Such a situation would require monitoring and would need a comparison of daily 'balances' over a number of days. Similarly, in a patient who has accumulated fluid overload, perhaps because of heart failure, the nurse will be looking for a negative balance at the end of the day. This will indicate how effective therapy, such as diuretic medication, has been.

Normal (maintenance) daily fluid requirements for an adult are approximately 1 mL/kg/hr. This amount would be increased in fever and to account for losses such as wound drainage.

Fluid balance charts (FBCs)

Different healthcare establishments use different charts, and methods for monitoring fluid balance will differ depending on how the chart is used. The chart may start and finish at 07.00 hrs, allowing the next day's fluid requirements to be set first thing in the morning. Other establishments use charts that start and finish around midnight, arguing that the least activity to do with fluid intake and output in most patients is at this time and so it is a sensible time to do the totting up. It also means that the chart needs to be dated only once.

Other differences may be in how the amounts are totalled and when the balance calculation is made. For example, there may be a column that allows for a running total of both input and output and running balance, or the chart may be balanced only once a day. Considering the body's responses to fluids, a daily balance is generally adequate. However, some patients may require more frequent recording of balance, such as individuals with poor renal function, patients losing significant amounts of blood or other body fluids, or those with a brain injury that prevents the normal homeostatic processes from occurring. Some units/wards require IV fluids to be added in only on completion; others add them in when they are put up and subtract the amount remaining at the end of the calculation period.

Good practice point

It is important that you understand the fluid balance chart recording process adopted where you work, as errors can arise through different interpretations of the data. Accurate recording of kept fluid balance charts can be very informative.

Worked example 9.1: fluid balance chart

Figure 9.1 is a fluid balance chart for John Smith, who weighs 73 kg. There are several things to do with the numbers on the chart that you should understand and that require you to apply your nursing knowledge. The numbers can tell us more than just the fluid balance; they can help us plan care. All volumes are in millilitres but this is not indicated on the chart, which is common practice.

First, it is important to note how the balance for the 24-hour period has been calculated. In Figure 9.1, the amounts are totalled both by *row* and by *column*, which provides an automatic check on the accuracy of calculations. Note that the numbers have been kept neatly so that accurate adding and subtraction is easier. When totalling fluid balance charts, it is sensible to check your calculations using

Figure 9.1 Fluid balance chart

Source: Based on that used by Royal Wolverhampton NHS Trust with their permission

Name: John Smith					Hospital No. 1234567			Date: Friday 7th March 20XX		
Time	Oral	Intravenous 1	Intravenous 2	Intravenous 3	Other	**Total IN**	Urine	Vomit	Other	**Total OUT**	Balance –ve/+ve
0100		Dext 5% (100)									
0200		N. Saline (1000)				100					+100
0300											
0400											
0500											
0600											
0700	60					60					+60
0800	25					25	320		Drain 100 red	420	–395
0900							100			100	–100
1000		Dext 5% (1000)				1000					+1000
1100	50					50					+50
1200							150			150	–150
1300	100					100					+100
1400	25					25					+25
1500							200	140		340	–340
1600	90					90			Drain 50 pink	50	+40
1700											
1800	25	N. Saline (500)				1025	270			270	+755
1900							100				–100
2000	50					50					+50
2100											
2200	75					75	230		Drain 10 clear	240	–165
2300											
2400						500					+500
Total	500	2600				3100	1170	340	160	1670	+1430
Daily Total						3100			+800=	2470	+630

a calculator. With the inbuilt checking mechanisms through the row and column totals mentioned above, use of a calculator may make the task quicker.

Observe how the intravenous fluids on this chart have not been added in to the input total until the patient has actually received them, but the amount 'put up' is in brackets. There is an entry at the beginning of the chart of 100 mL Dextrose 5%. This appears as the amount left to be infused when the previous day's chart ended at midnight.

In the final row of the chart you will see the amount +800 printed, which is to be added to the total output. This is a figure representing the insensible (not easily measured) loss of fluid that occurs through expiration, evaporation of sweat and fluid content of normal faeces.

What things might this chart indicate to us?

- Look at the intake, which is the recommended amount for his weight. If a patient is able to drink as normally as this suggests, then IV fluids may not be necessary.
- Look at the output. Urine output is not abnormal but it is less than would be expected from the amount of intake. It may be that Mr Smith was slightly dehydrated and is compensating. You could check the previous day's chart to confirm.
- The amount of wound drainage is tailing off. This might indicate that it is time for the drain to be shortened or removed.
- If you look carefully, you may also notice that the patient appears to vomit a small amount after an oral intake (amount entered as 25 mL). This might suggest that the small amount is taken with some oral medication and that the vomiting is associated with this. He does not appear to vomit after meals or other drinks. This is something worth mentioning and investigating, as his medication may need to be changed.

While this book does not cover nursing care, this information from the fluid balance chart illustrates how much you can learn from numbers and how important it is to calculate correctly and to keep accurate records, across your nursing care.

Sometimes patients may be given fluid that is expected to be returned – for example, as bladder irrigation or peritoneal dialysis fluid. This may be entered on a separate chart or may be integrated with the normal fluid balance chart. The calculation of fluid balance for such patients requires keeping a careful record of how much fluid is being exchanged.

Worked example 9.2: fluid balance chart including irrigation fluid

Mr Vale is a 60-year-old man who has had a transurethral prostatectomy and requires continuous bladder irrigation. The normal fluid balance chart has been adapted for his case. An extract from it is shown below.

Name: Robin Vale				Hospital No. 2468102				Date: Friday 7th March 20XX			
Time	Oral	Intravenous 1	Intravenous 2	~~Intravenous~~ 3 Irrigation	Other	Total IN	Urine	Vomit	Other Bladder Drain	Total OUT	Balance −ve/+ve
0800	120	5% Dext 100		N.Saline 250		470			600 br.red	600	
0900		IV Dise									
1000	100			N.Saline 1000		1100			600 red	600	
1100	180					180					
1200	200					200			500 clear pk	500	

In the remainder of the day there was further fluid intake and output. The final totals for the day were:

Total	2100	100		3750		5950			5150		
Daily Total						5950			+800=	5950	0

The calculations are the same as for any other fluid balance chart. We need to add up the total amount going in and subtract the amount coming out, remembering to allow for insensible losses. Note that as with the IV fluids in the earlier examples of fluid balance charts, the irrigation fluid has not been recorded in the total column until it has all gone in.

The difference here is that we can only account for urine output by looking at the difference in totals between the column headed 'irrigation' and that headed 'bladder drainage'. In this example, the amount of irrigation fluid used was 3750 mL and the bladder drainage was 5150 mL. Therefore, urine output must have been the total bladder drainage *minus* the amount of irrigation fluid. In other words:

5150 − 3750 = 1400 mL.

Dialysis

Patients with severe renal failure need to have their kidney function replaced by some other means. This artificial process of 'cleansing' the blood is called *dialysis*.

Haemo-dialysis works on the principle of taking the patient's blood out of the body and circulating it across a membrane where unwanted elements are extracted by osmosis or diffusion and withdrawn from the blood, while required substances are retained and/or can be added. The blood is then reintroduced to the body.

Haemo-filtration is another method of managing renal failure in which a semi-permeable membrane allows a filtrate of plasma to be excreted and the losses replaced by intravenous solutions.

An alternative is *peritoneal dialysis*, a process involving the introduction of dialysis fluid into the peritoneum where the body's own capacity for osmosis will exchange electrolytes which are lacking for those products which the body needs to excrete.

The fluid itself is the transport medium for the waste products and so it is essential to keep an accurate record of just how much goes in and how much comes out, as well as keeping a normal fluid balance record for these patients. Sometimes the patient, particularly in paediatrics, is nursed on a weigh bed, which allows for constant monitoring of their weight, which is an additional check of how much fluid is being lost or retained.

Worked example 9.3: peritoneal dialysis

Mrs Lake has begun continuous peritoneal dialysis and her weight is being recorded hourly, along with a record of the fluid balance relating to her dialysis. An extract from her chart is shown below. Note that the cumulative total is a running total of the amount of fluid lost or gained at each time of entry.

Weight (kg)	Solution IN (fill time 10 min)			Solution OUT (drain time 20 min)			Difference per cycle	Cumulative difference (mL)
	Start	Finish	Vol (mL)	Start	Finish	Vol (mL)		
51.5	09.00	09.10	2000	10.00	10.20	2100	−100	−100
51.25	10.20	10.30	2000	11.30	11.50	1950	+50	−50
51.67	11.50	12.00	2000	13.00	13.20	1830	+170	+120
51.61	13.20	13.30	2000	14.30	14.50	2150	−150	−30
50.4	14.50	15.00	2000	16.00	16.20	2300	−300	−330
51.45	16.20	16.30	2000	17.30	17.50	1740	+260	−70
						Sub-total		−70

By recording the loss or gain at each cycle and totalling this column, we have an instant check of our cumulative total.

Infant fluids

Babies and young children are at greater risk of fluid imbalance due to their immature kidneys, and being less able to help themselves to fluids when thirsty.

Newborn babies need about 150 mL per kg of body weight per day; therefore, the total amount calculated needs to be divided by 6 or 8 to administer as 4- or 3-hourly feeds respectively. For example, if a newborn is fed every 4 hours, the total daily fluid intake should be divided by 6 (because 6 feeds × 4 hours = 24 hours).

In UK maternity and children's hospitals, this may be calculated by the dietician and sent up from the milk kitchen already prepared. However, as the person administering the feed, you must be sure that the amount is correct for the individual baby by doing the usual checks.

Worked example 9.4: Infant feeds

How much feed would you expect to give to a 3.28 kg baby aged one week? First, calculate the recommended daily amount for the baby:

150 mL per kg of body weight = 150 × 3.28 = 492 mL

For 4-hourly feeds, divide by 6:

492 ÷ 6 = 82 mL per feed

For 3-hourly feeds, divide by 8:

492 ÷ 8 = 61.5 mL per feed

Then *check* – is this what has been prepared and is it a sensible amount for the size of baby?

Infant feeds and fluid balance

Children require fluid input in volume related to their weight. Correct calculation of fluid balance is particularly vital in children, especially those with cardiac, renal or liver function problems who may have restricted intake. Pre-term babies and those receiving phototherapy may require additional fluids, while enterally fed infants will often require higher fluid allowance for optimal growth. Feeds have to be taken into account and *all* fluid measured, including drug volumes.

The type of calculation, which the nurse may need to make, is to work out what volume of maintenance feed (fluid containing nutrients) can be given within the total fluid allowance. This allows the dietician to make up the content appropriately. There may be slight variations in local guidelines for recommended mL/hr/kg. Typical amounts are shown in Table 9.1. The calculation may involve percentages, addition, and subtraction.

Neat charts make addition of columns much easier and reduce the risk of calculation errors. Using your calculator to add up totals is fine, but you need to cross-check regularly to a running total.

Table 9.1 is to be used to calculate appropriate fluid requirements. Fluids should be prescribed as a percentage of normal maintenance rather than mL/kg. For example, a child weighing 40 kg being restricted to 50% of normal should receive 40 mL/hr. Pre-term babies and those receiving phototherapy may require additional fluids. Enterally fed infants will often require a higher fluid allowance for optimum growth (up to 150% of values given in Table 9.1).

Different NHS Trusts use different proformas, but the nurse needs to be aware of how to fill these in using the local conventions.

Worked example 9.5: bolus feeds

A 6-month-old infant weighing 6.7 kg is to have five bottle feeds a day. She also has a combination of intravenous (IV) drugs prescribed, which amount to 12.5 mL every 6 hours. How much feed can she have per bottle?

Table 9.1   Maintenance of intravenous fluid requirements

Weight (kg)	100% Maintenance mL/hour
3	13
4	17
6	25
8	33
10	42
12	46
14	50
16	54
18	58
20	63
30	71
40	79
50	88
60	96

Note: Calculated using the Holliday-Segar Method. Details can be found at: Holliday, M.A., Segar, W.E. (1957) The maintenance need for water in parenteral fluid therapy, *Pediatrics*, 19(5): 823–832.

First, calculate the recommended daily amount of fluid for a baby of this weight:

150 mL per kg of body weight = 150 × 6.7 = 1005 mL

Next, calculate how much fluid she is receiving in IV drugs per day:

12.5 mL every 6 hours is the same as 4 × 12.5 mL over 24 hours = 4 × 12.5 = 50 mL

Subtract the total volume of drugs from the fluid allowance to get the remainder that can be given as feed:

1005 – 50 = 955 mL

For the amount per feed, divide this by number of feeds per day (5):

955 ÷ 5 = 191 mL

This is approximately 190 mL per bottle. *Check*: is this a sensible amount for a baby's bottle feed?

Worked example 9.6: continuous feeding

A child weighing 12 kg is prescribed 75% of maintenance fluids over 24 hours. He is being fed continuously by a nasogastric tube attached to a feed pump. Approximately, how much of the hourly intake should be fed?

According to local policy, 100% maintenance IV fluid requirements for a 12 kg child is 46 mL/hr (see Table 9.1). So what is 75% of 46 mL/hr?

First, do a rough *estimate*:

75% is the same as $\dfrac{3}{4}$, so the amount must be less than 46 (the whole amount) but more than 23 (which is half):

$$75\% = \frac{75}{100}$$

$$75\% \text{ of } 46 = \frac{75}{100} \times 46\,\text{mL/hr}$$

Divide the top and bottom by 25 to give:

$$\frac{\cancel{75}^{3}}{\cancel{100}_{4}} \times \frac{46}{1}$$

Then multiply across to get $\dfrac{138}{4}$.

Use the percentage key on your calculator instead of dividing by 100 if you wish, but always check your answer against the estimate.

The answer is 34.5. So the child should be receiving a total of 34.5 mL per hour.

But when you look at the prescription sheet, you realize that continuous infusions of various drugs amount to 5 mL/hr and antibiotics add another 15 mL every 6 hours. Taking these into account, what is the amount of feed which can be given per hour?

First, *calculate* the total volume of prescribed drugs/fluid per hour:

IV infusions = 5 mL/hr
Antibiotics = 15 mL in 6 hours = $15 \div 6 = 2.5$ mL/hr
Total volume of infusions/drugs per hour is 7.5 mL

Therefore, the child can be given a feed of

$$
\begin{array}{r}
3 \quad 4 \quad . \quad 5 \quad 0 \\
- \quad\quad 7 \quad . \quad 5 \quad\quad \\
\hline
2 \quad 7 \quad . \quad 0 \quad 0 \quad \text{mL/hr}
\end{array}
$$

Check that this is a sensible amount.

Chapter summary

We have seen how to deal with the common types of calculations you are likely to encounter in general situations. As pointed out, there are some areas of nursing, such as intensive care and high dependency units, where more complicated calculations are required. The next chapter is intended to cover the calculations you may come across in these specialist areas.

10 Specialized calculations: percentages, ratios, neonates, and body surface area

This chapter covers:

- Calculations involving percentages and ratios
- Neonates/PICU
- Calculations based on body surface area (BSA)

Percentages and ratios

The concepts of percentage and ratio were covered briefly in Chapter 3. The calculations are not difficult, but many people have trouble understanding what the numbers mean and so can make errors relating to magnitude, which may have serious consequences. When doing calculations involving percentages, ratios or proportion, the golden rule of estimation should always be applied.

 Good practice point

Percentage solutions used in healthcare generally indicate *grams of solid dissolved in 100 mL of solution*. A commonly used intravenous fluid is 5% dextrose. Remember that percentage means 'in a hundred' and 5% is the same as the fraction $\frac{5}{100}$. So, the 5% in *5% dextrose* indicates that in every 100 mL of the solution, there are 5 g of dextrose, because generally 1 mL water weighs (and is therefore equivalent to) 1 g in weight.

Worked example 10.1: percentage (I)

We want to know how much dextrose is in a one-litre (1000 mL) bag of 5% dextrose. In other words, what is 5% of 1000 mL?

$$\frac{1000}{1} \times \frac{5}{100}$$

We can simplify by dividing top and bottom by 100 to get:

$$10 \times 5 = 50 \text{ g}$$

Thus, there are 50 g dextrose in a litre bag of 5% dextrose.

Expressing fractions as percentages (and vice versa)

To express a fraction as a percentage, multiply by 100. Thus, $\frac{1}{2}$ expressed as a percentage is $\frac{100}{2}$ or 50%. It might be helpful to show the stages of multiplying by 100, and how we got to 50 as the actual percentage:

$$\frac{1}{2} \times \frac{100}{1} = \frac{100}{2} = 50$$

To express a percentage as a fraction or decimal, divide by 100. Thus, 25% is the same as $\frac{25}{100}$, which simplifies to $\frac{1}{4}$ or 0.25.

Worked example 10.2: percentage (II)

A local anaesthetic cream contains 2.5% lidocaine. How much lidocaine is there in a 5 g tube? So, what is 2.5% of 5?

Calculate: $\frac{2.5}{100} \times \frac{5}{1}$

Multiply across the fraction to get $\frac{12.5}{100}$ and then divide by 100 by moving the decimal point

$$= 0.125 \text{ g}$$

Thus, a 5 g tube of the cream contains 0.125 g of lidocaine.

Worked example 10.3: percentage (III)

Chlorhexidine 0.05% can be used for cleansing wounds. What is the strength of this solution in mg/mL?

We know that percentage solutions used in healthcare indicate grams of solid dissolved in 100 mL of solution, so 0.05% indicates 0.05 g of chlorhexidine in 100 mL.

If 100 mL = 0.05 g (it will be easier to change this to 50 mg at this point), then:

$$1 \text{ mL} = \frac{50}{100} \text{mg} = 0.5 \text{ mg}$$

Thus, the strength of a 0.05% solution is 0.5 mg/mL.

The following two worked examples show how percentage calculations might be used in situations not related to medication. It is still important to understand how percentages work in relation to other parts of your work.

Worked example 10.4: percentage (iv)

Percentages are often used in reports. For example, a local authority reports a Caesarean section (CS) rate of 24% of births in 2016. If the total number of births under that authority in 2016 was 30,642, how many were delivered by CS? The calculation is:

24% of 30,642

$$\frac{24}{100} \times 30{,}642$$

With numbers this large, it may be easier to simplify first, before multiplying across, so simplify by dividing both figures by 100:

$$= 24 \times 306.42$$
$$= 7354.08$$

As this number applies to births, we can sensibly disregard the .08 and conclude that there were 7354 Caesarean sections in this local authority in 2016.

Worked example 10.5: percentage (v)

We could equally work out the percentage rate if we knew the total number of deliveries and the number that were Caesarean sections. Thus, 5000 CS deliveries in a total of 31,500 deliveries would mean a percentage rate of:

$$\frac{5000}{31{,}500} \times \frac{100}{1} \% = 15.9\%$$

Ratios and proportion

One source of confusion (and potential error) in medication calculations relates to the use of solutions whose strength is given as a proportion or ratio. Common examples are wound dressings and skin preparations such as potassium permanganate 1 in 1000.

To understand the strength of a solution, we should recognize what this means. 1 in 1000 is the same as $\dfrac{1}{1000}$ or 0.1%, which means one part of active ingredient in 1000 parts of the solution.

To convert a percentage to a proportion, change it into a fraction first.

Worked example 10.6: proportions

What is a 0.02% solution as a proportion?

0.02% solution = 0.02 g of solute in 100 mL of solution

To show this as a proportion, we need to express it as a fraction with a whole number on the top:

$$0.02\% = \frac{0.02}{100}$$

To convert the 0.02 to a whole number, we multiply by 100. So that we do not change the value of the fraction, we do the same to the denominator, resulting in:

$$\frac{2}{10{,}000} \text{ or, when simplified, } \frac{1}{5000}$$

Thus we can say that a 0.02% solution is the same as 1 in 5000 solution.

Many things that require dilution, such as milk powders, have specific instructions as to the number of measures of powder to use with a specific volume of liquid, and so are easy to calculate. However, the final result should always be checked to confirm it is sensible.

Worked example 10.7: dilution of solutions

Potassium permanganate is available as a 0.1% or 1 in 1000 solution, but for use as a wet dressing, the BNF suggests further dilution with water to 1 in 10,000.

Let us suppose that we need 100 mL of solution.

- *Estimate* – the required solution is 10 times weaker than the stock available, and so we are going to need one-tenth of the stock solution. In 100 mL, this would be 10 mL. By estimating, we can see that we do not actually need to do a calculation, but the calculation is detailed to illustrate the principle.
- Then, *calculate* how much active ingredient would be in 100 mL of the required 1 in 10,000 solution.

    1 in 10,000 = 0.01%

Remember, 0.01 g in 100 mL, so we require 0.01 g of active ingredient. To get this amount from the stock solution (0.1% or 0.1 g in 100 mL), we can use the methods of dosage calculation used throughout the book.

Applying the NHS1 formula:

$$\frac{\text{what you need}}{\text{what you have}} \times \frac{\text{stock volume}}{1} = \text{dose in mL.}$$

Now, substitute values into the equation:

$$\frac{0.01}{0.1} \times \frac{100}{1} \text{mL} = 10 \, \text{mL}$$

So, we require 10 mL of the stock solution and 90 mL of water to produce the required strength (1 in 10,000).

Neonates and paediatric intensive care

In high dependency areas, such as paediatric intensive care units (PICU), children may be given continuous infusions of a variety of drugs via syringe drivers. Accurate calculations and checking, regarding all aspects of the prescription and delivery, are vitally important and this is one of the things a nurse will do when taking over the care of a child from another at the change of shift as well as when a prescription is new, or the syringe requires changing. You must be certain that you agree with the set-up that you are 'inheriting', as the accountability for the child's care passes to you at this point. Nomograms are not normally used in children's units and so calculation skills are vital.

Many pharmaceutical companies provide clinical trials data relating to safe drug dosages for paediatric patients in milligrams per kilogram (mg/kg) of body weight. Based on this information, the paediatric dose can be determined by multiplying the weight of the patient (in kilograms) by the prescribed number of milligrams of drug per kilogram (which may be reported per dose or per day).

When calculating doses for paediatric drugs, the following equation may be used:

Dose required = body weight (kg) × recommended dose (mg/kg/day)

Worked example 10.8: Inotropes in children

A newborn baby (3 kg) who has had surgery to correct a congenital heart defect requires inotropic support in the form of a continuous infusion.

Name of drug	Amount	Route	Frequency
DOBUTAMINE	Solution made up as 90 mg in total volume of 50 mL	IV	1 mL/hr

The label on the ampoule reads: Dobutamine 50 mg/mL

The recommended diluent is 5% glucose for dilution to a concentration of not more than 5 mg/mL. The recommended dosage for a newborn baby is 2–10 microgram/kg/min.

This calculation is going to have several stages, but let's stick to the principles we have used throughout the book. We can use these first to calculate how to make up the prescribed solution.

- *Extract* the relevant information from the prescription:
  Drug = 90 mg dobutamine.

The diluent is 50% glucose, already made up as such (thus the 50% is just a part of the labelling and does not come into the calculation). Made up to 50 mL means we will need 50 mL of diluent MINUS the volume of dobutamine.

- *Check the prescription* – we'll leave this until we have calculated how to produce the required solution.
- *Check* that the drug is available in the same units as the prescription:
  Yes, both are milligrams.
- *Estimate* an approximate answer:
  We need 90 mg. The drug is available as 50 mg/mL and so we can estimate an amount of more than 1 mL but less than 2 mL.
- *Calculate*
  Applying the NHS1 formula:

$$\frac{\text{what you need}}{\text{what you have}} \times \frac{\text{stock volume}}{1} = \text{dose in mL.}$$

Substitute the known values to get your answer:

$$\frac{90}{50} \times 1 = 1.8 \text{ mL}$$

- *Check this answer* against your approximation.

We had estimated more than 1 mL and less than 2 mL, so this is a sensible answer to have got.

The final step to preparing the solution is to look at the dilution instructions, which were:

Solution made up as 90 mg in total volume of 50 mL.

We need 1.8 mL (90 mg) of the drug to be made up to a total volume of 50 mL and so we require:

(50 – 1.8) mL of diluents = 48.2 mL

Therefore, to make up the 50 mL of solution to be infused, we need 1.8 mL of dobutamine in 48.2 mL of 5% glucose.

- *Check this is safe for the patient*:
  Would this dose be right for a newborn baby?
  The recommended dose is 2–10 microgram/kg/min.
  We need to work this through as a separate calculation.
- *Check* that the drug is available in the same units as the prescription:
  NO: the drug is available in mg/mL and we are looking at a recommended rate involving micrograms.

To work out whether the prescription fits with the recommended dose and rate for a newborn, we need to calculate:

- how many micrograms are contained in 1 mL of the solution prescribed
- how many micrograms of drug is right for this weight of baby at the rate prescribed.

We have made up a solution of 90 mg dobutamine in 50 mL, so what would that be in 1 mL?

If 50 mL = 90 mg,

then $1 \text{ mL} = \dfrac{90}{50} \text{ mg}$.

To change this to micrograms, multiply by 1000:

$$\frac{90}{50} \times 1000 = 90 \times 20 = 1800 \text{ micrograms}$$

So, we have a solution that contains 1800 micrograms per mL.

The delivery rate is 1 mL/hr, which is what we will set the syringe driver to deliver and this will give the baby 1800 microgram of dobutamine per hour. Is this a safe amount for the baby?

Recommended amount is 2–10 microgram/kg/min.

We still need to calculate the rate of delivery in minutes to be able to compare it with the recommended dose:

1800 microgram per hour is how many microgram per minute?

- *Estimate or use a common-sense check.* Would the amount delivered in a minute be more or less than that delivered in an hour? The answer is, of course, less. So we need to divide by 60 to change the rate from hourly to per minute:

1800 micrograms (mcg) per hour $= \dfrac{1800}{60}$ mcg per minute

$= 30$ mcg per minute

Is this a safe amount for the baby? Remember, the recommended amount is 2–10 microgram/kg/min. The baby weighs 3 kg, so the maximum amount for him would be 10×3 microgram per minute:

= 30 mcg per minute

This is exactly what we have calculated as being the amount delivered by the prescription and so we can safely go ahead with the delivery as instructed.

Calculations based on body surface area (BSA)

In children (or adults) who are either extremely underweight or overweight for their age, dose by weight can be an unreliable method of calculating a therapeutic dose. Body surface area (BSA) gives a more accurate basis for calculating doses, as it is a better indicator of metabolic processes. BSAs are calculated using standard tables, nomograms or a formula that provides an estimate of BSA based on the weight of the child (Table 10.1).

Table 10.1 Formula for BSA estimation

Weight range	Formula for estimation of BSA
1–5 kg	M^2 BSA = $(0.05 \times$ kg wt$)$ + 0.05
6–10 kg	M^2 BSA = $(0.04 \times$ kg wt$)$ + 0.10
11–20 kg	M^2 BSA = $(0.03 \times$ kg wt$)$ + 0.20
21–70 kg	M^2 BSA = $(0.02 \times$ kg wt$)$ + 0.40

Source: Rudolph, A.M. (1982) *Paediatrics*, 17th edn. Norwalk, CT: Appleton-Century-Crofts.

A table based on ideal body weights of children from newborn (full term) to 12 years is provided in the back of the BNF and through the BNF online [https://www.bnf.org/]. The formula given there is based on the assumption that the BSA of a 70 kg adult is 1.8 m^2 and looks like this:

$$\text{Approximate dose} = \frac{\text{BSA of child (m}^2)}{1.8 \text{ m}^2} \times \text{adult dose}$$

Thus, starting with an adult dose of 125 mg, find the dose for a child with a BSA of 0.62 m^2.

- *Applying the formula*

$$\text{Approximate dose} = \frac{0.62}{1.8} \times 125 \text{ mg}$$

- *Estimate* an answer by looking at the numbers and rounding where sensible:

$$\frac{0.6}{1.8} = \frac{6}{18} = \frac{1}{3}$$

one-third of 123 or $(\frac{1}{3} \times 123) = 41$

So, we can estimate that the answer should be around 41 mg. The actual calculation gives us 43 mg.

Chapter summary

The administration of drugs in the paediatric setting is a complex and specialist area. It is based mainly on body weight, although certain drugs are prescribed and administered based on body surface area. However, BSA is not routinely used by nurses for calculating medication dosage.

Significant differences in the distribution, metabolism, and therapeutic index (TI) of drugs between adults and children mean that practitioners should always use extreme caution when prescribing or administering drugs to children, as even small differences or errors can have potentially life-threatening consequences.

11 Specialized calculations: complex prescriptions, nomograms, and parenteral nutrition

This chapter covers:

- Complex prescriptions
- Use of nomograms
- Parenteral nutrition

Complex prescriptions

Patients requiring intensive care are often on a variety of drugs that are part of a life support system. The calculations required to ensure that correct dosages are received can be quite difficult, as they can involve several different measurements, including the patient's weight, strength of solution, and rate of delivery. Inotropic drugs, which are used to increase the force of cardiac contraction, are a good example of this. Due to their potency, they are generally administered via a central venous line, rather than a peripheral line, and delivery is always controlled through a delivery device such as an electronic syringe pump or driver.

Worked example 11.1: complex prescriptions

An adult male weighing 80 kg requires dobutamine at a rate of 5 microgram/kg/min. You will need to understand how much to deliver, how much this is per minute, and whether this is in line with the recommended dose.

The prescription is:

Name of drug	Amount	Route	Frequency
DOBUTAMINE	Solution made up in dextrose 5% as 3 mg/kg in total volume of 50 mL	IV via central line	5 mL/hr

The recommended adult dose is 2–10 microgram/kg/min.

The label on the ampoule reads: | Dobutamine 250 mg in 20 mL |

- *Extract* the relevant information from the prescription:
  Drug = 3 mg/kg dobutamine.

The diluent is 5% dextrose (the 5% is part of the labelling and does not come into the calculation).

- *Check the prescription.*
  The rate prescribed is within the recommended guidelines.
  If made up as directed, how much dobutamine is needed and will this give the correct amount for our patient?

Stage 1: Make up solution

- *Check* that the drug is available in the same units as the prescription:
  Yes, both are milligrams.
- *Estimate dose:*
  Weight 80 kg × 3 mg = 240 mg.
  Dobutamine is supplied as 250 mg in a 20 mL ampoule.
  240 mg is close to 250 and so we will need just under 20 mL.
- *Calculate using your chosen method.*
  We can apply the formula:

$$\text{Volume required} = \frac{\text{strength prescribed}}{\text{strength available}} \times \frac{\text{volume of stock}}{1}$$

Substitute the known values to get your answer:

$$\frac{240}{250} \times \frac{20}{1} = \frac{96}{5} = 19.2 \text{ mL.}$$

- *Check this answer* against your approximation.

To make up the required solution to a total of 50 mL, we have to add (50 – 19.2) mL of diluent. We will use dextrose 5%:

= 30.8 mL dextrose 5%

We now have 50 mL of a solution containing 240 mg dobutamine.

Stage 2: Check that this is safe to give at the rate prescribed

The prescription is for delivery to be 5 mL/hr. How much dobutamine is this per minute?

240 mg in 50 mL is equivalent to 24 mg in 5 mL of this solution.

24 mg delivered over 60 minutes means $\dfrac{24}{60} = \dfrac{2}{5}$ or 0.4 mg per minute

0.4 mg = 400 micrograms

The prescribed rate of 5 mL/hr will deliver 400 microgram/minute.

- *Check* that this will deliver the required amount of 5 microgram/kg/min.
  At weight 80 kg, 5 microgram/kg = 400 micrograms.
  Hence, the prescription is safe to give.

Nomograms

As we have seen in the previous section, as well as in Chapter 10, the calculations involved in inotropic doses and rate of administration can be quite complicated. To reduce the chance of error, many adult high dependency and intensive care units use *nomograms* or nomogram conversion charts to make certain frequently needed calculations easier for the medical and nursing staff. They are less common for children's nursing because of the small amounts used and the huge range of sizes among children.

Nomograms are complicated graphs that are usually converted to tables for use with drugs that are given by infusion on a microgram/kilogram/minute (mcg/kg/min) basis. These are typically vasoactive or cardiac drugs such as dobutamine, dopamine, adrenaline, noradrenaline (all inotropes), and glyceryl trinitrate (GTN), which acts as a vasodilator.

We will use nomograms for dopamine to show how they can be constructed in two main ways:

Method 1. The dose of dopamine is diluted into a *variable* volume of diluent (usually 0.9% saline) so that 1 mcg/kg/min is achieved by setting the syringe pump at 1 mL/hour.

Method 2. The dose of dopamine is diluted into a *fixed* volume of diluent and the syringe pump rate adjusted to give the appropriate mcg/kg/min.

Worked example 11.2: dopamine nomogram – method 1

The dose of dopamine is diluted into a *variable* volume of diluent, so that 1 mcg/kg/min is achieved by setting the syringe pump at 1 mL/hr:

- The patient weighs 70 kg. To achieve 1 mcg/kg/min, we need to deliver 70 (70 × 1) mcg per minute.
- The syringe pump setting allows for mL per hour, so we need to convert our minutes to hours by multiplying by 60.
- 70 mcg per minute will be 70 × 60 mcg per hour, or 4200 mcg/hr.

Just take a minute to check that this is sensible.

For 1 mcg/kg/min to equal 1 mL/hr, the concentration of dopamine needs to be 4200 mcg per mL.

The label on the ampoule reads:

> Dopamine Hydrochloride
> 200 mg in 5 mL

Dopamine is supplied as 200 mg in 5 mL, but remember that we need micrograms, so first we need to change 200 mg into micrograms (mcg):

1 mg = 1000 mcg
200 mg = 200,000 mcg

and so, the 5 mL ampoule contains 200,000 mcg of dopamine.

What volume of diluent (v) do we need to dilute this to 4200 mcg/mL? In other words, in what volume will 200,000 mcg equal 4200 mcg in 1mL?

Set up the equation:

$$\frac{200,000}{v} = \frac{4200}{1}$$

By dividing both sides by 4200 and multiplying both sides by v, we get:

$$\frac{200,000}{4200} = v$$

Simplify by dividing both the top and bottom by 200 to get:

$$v = \frac{1000}{21} = 47.6$$

Rounded to the nearest whole number, the volume we need is 48 mL. This means we have to dilute the dopamine to 48 mL of solution to give 4200 mcg of dopamine per mL. As dopamine is supplied in 5 mL ampoules, we need (48 – 5 =) 43 mL of diluent.

As you can appreciate, this is a complex calculation and it would be tedious to have to do it for each patient. Therefore, in most intensive care environments, tabulations of nomograms like the one shown in Table 11.1 are available.

In practice, the chart would have weight increasing in 1 kg intervals. Using this table to prepare the solution means that a rate of 2 mL/hr will deliver 2 mcg/kg/min, while 3 mL/hr will deliver 3 mcg/kg/min, and so on.

Note that for a patient of 50 kg, the total volume exceeds the 60 mL capacity of the syringes normally used in syringe pumps/drivers. In this case, it is considered

Table 11.1 Extract from tabulated nomogram for dopamine (method 1)

mcg/kg/min	Patient's weight	Dopamine dose (mg)	Dopamine volume (mL)	Diluent volume (mL)	Total volume (mL)	Pump rate (mL/hr)
1	50	200	5	62	67	1
1	60	200	5	51	56	1
1	70	200	5	43	48	1
1	80	200	5	37	42	1
1	90	200	5	32	37	1

good practice to halve both the amount of dopamine and the total volume, resulting in 100 mg dopamine (2.5 mL) diluted in 31 mL of diluent to a total volume of 33.5 mL.

Worked example 11.3: dopamine nomogram – method 2

The dose of dopamine is diluted into a *fixed* volume of diluent and the syringe pump rate adjusted to give the appropriate mcg/kg/min:

- A 5 mL ampoule of dopamine contains 200 mg. This is diluted with 45 mL of diluent to a constant volume of 50 mL.
- The concentration of dopamine is now $\dfrac{200}{50}$ or 4 mg/mL.
- 4 mg = 4000 mcg and so this is equivalent to 4000 mcg/mL.

Using this solution, at what rate will we need to set the syringe pump/driver to deliver 1 mcg/kg/min to a 70 kg person?

1 mcg/kg/min for a 70 kg person = 70 mcg/min or 70 × 60 mcg/hr = 4200 mcg/hr

If the concentration is 4000 mcg/mL, what rate must the pump be set at?

- *Estimate.* We need just over 4000 mcg per hour, so the rate of delivery should be just over 1 mL/hr.
- *Calculate.* The calculation may be best explained by going back to one of the methods suggested for straightforward drug dosage calculations and finding what rate in mL/hr is equivalent to 1 mcg/hr so that we can then multiply up to 4200 mcg/hr.

We know that 1 mL/hr = 4000 mcg/hr. Therefore,

$\dfrac{1}{4000}$ mL/hr = 1 mcg/hr

Thus $\dfrac{1}{4000}$ × 4200 mL/hr = 4200 mcg/hr.

Simplified this becomes $\dfrac{42}{40}$ mL/hr = 4200 mcg/hr,

or 1.05 mL/hr will deliver 4200 mcg/hr.

Hence, the pump should be set at 1.05 mL/hr.

- *Check against the estimate*: just over 1 mL/hr was our estimate.

As with method 1, repetitive calculations of this type can be tedious and the complicated nature of the calculation means that errors are more likely to be made. Hence a tabulated nomogram like the one in Table 11.2 is very useful and also allows for higher doses of dopamine to be calculated.

Table 11.2 Extract from tabulated nomogram for dopamine (method 2)

Patient's weight (kg)	mcg/ kg/min	Dopamine dose (mg)	Dopamine volume (mL)	Diluent volume (mL)	Total volume (mL)	Pump rate (mL/hr)
50	1	200	5	45	50	0.75
	2	200	5	45	50	1.5
	4	200	5	45	50	3.0
60	1	200	5	45	50	0.9
	2	200	5	45	50	1.8
	4	200	5	45	50	3.6
70	1	200	5	45	50	1.05
	2	200	5	45	50	2.1
	4	200	5	45	50	4.2
80	1	200	5	45	50	1.2
	2	200	5	45	50	2.4
	4	200	5	45	50	4.8

Parenteral nutrition

Parenteral nutrition is administered to a patient when their nutritional requirements cannot be met because of increased metabolic demand, or because of impaired digestion or absorption processes. The procedure involves administering commercially available products or specially formulated pharmacy preparations. This might be via a central or peripheral vein, but in most cases nutrients are delivered directly to the gastrointestinal (GI) tract by means of a percutaneous endoscopic gastrostomy (PEG) tube.

The flow of PEG feeding is normally controlled by an automated infusion pump (see Chapter 8 for more on infusion pumps). These automatic devices are similar to those used for drug infusions, whereby a pre-determined flow rate can be set. To check that the infusion is being administered at a suitable rate, it is important to be able to determine the finish time, given the start time and the flow rate.

The basic formula is given below.

$$\text{Protocol time (hours)} = \frac{\text{volume of infusion}}{\text{flow rate}}$$

If the infusion has to run for a significant number of hours, a break may be incorporated into the protocol. The length of this break must be added to the above formula to give the actual finish time.

$$\text{Protocol time (hours)} = \frac{\text{volume of infusion}}{\text{flow rate}} + \text{break time}$$

Worked example 11.4: parenteral nutrition

A patient has been prescribed 900 mL parenteral nutrition to be administered by PEG tube at a flow rate of 150 mL/hr. The infusion is scheduled to start at 07.30 hours with a 2-hour break mid-infusion. What time will the feed be completed?

- *Step 1*: Identify the equation you need.

$$\text{Protocol time (hours)} = \frac{\text{volume of infusion}}{\text{flow rate}} + \text{break time}$$

- *Step 2*: Substitute the volume of infusion (900 mL), flow rate (150 mL/hr), and break time (2 hours) into the equation and then simplify.

$$\text{Protocol time} = \frac{900 \text{ mL}}{150 \text{ mL/hr}} + 2 \text{ hours}$$

$$= \frac{\cancel{900}^{\,6}}{\cancel{150}_{\,1}} + 2 \text{ hours}$$

$$= 6 + 2 = 8 \text{ hours}$$

- *Step 3*: To determine the time at which the infusion should be terminated, add the protocol time to the start time.

Finish time = start time + protocol time.

In this case, the protocol time is 8 hours and the start time is 07.30 hours.

Finish time = 07.30 hours + 8 hours = 15.30 hours.

The answer is 15.30 hours.

Chapter summary

Some calculations in healthcare are complex and require practitioners to perform detailed and systematic numerical operations. It is important that professionals working in areas requiring such calculations are confident and regularly practise their skills to complete complex calculations.

Appendix A

Common abbreviations used in healthcare practice

	Abbreviation	Term in full	Definition, common examples of use and notes
Weight	g	gram	Measure of mass – drug dosages
	kg	kilogram	Base unit for mass = 1000 grams – weight of individuals
	mg	milligram	One-thousandth of a gram – drug dosages
	µg or mcg	microgram	One-millionth of a gram – drug dosages.Use of the abbreviation is *not recommended* because of similarity to mg. Write in full
Volume	cl	centilitre	One-hundredth of a litre
	L	litre	Base unit of volume. Note similarity to the number 1 and use with care
	mL or ml	millilitre	One-thousandth of a litre – liquid feeds, medication, drainage, urine and intravenous fluids
	vol	volume	Measure of capacity
Length	cm	centimetre	One-hundredth of a metre – baby's length and head circumference, central venous pressure (cm of water (H_2O))
	km	kilometre	One thousand metres – geographical distances
	m	metre	Base unit of length – height of individuals

	Abbreviation	Term in full	Definition, common examples of use and notes
	mm	millimetre	One-thousandth of a metre – blood pressure measurement (millimetres of mercury (mmHg))
	μm	micrometre	One-millionth of a metre. Used in measurement of cell size
Pressure	**B/P**	blood pressure	Measured in millimetres of mercury (mmHg)
	CVP	central venous pressure	Usually measured in centimetres of water (cm H_2O)
	PP	pulse pressure	The difference between the systolic and diastolic pressure readings and the pulse pressure is the pressure felt when you feel the pulse, which is generated by the force of the heart contracting. Pulse pressure is measured in millimetres of mercury (mmHg)
	paO$_2$	partial pressure of oxygen	Blood gas measurement
	Pa	Pascal	SI unit of pressure
Routes of administration	**ID**	Intradermal	Route of injection into the dermal layer
	IT	Intrathecal	Route of injection into the cerebro-spinal fluid within the dura
	IM	Intramuscular	Route of injection of drugs into the muscle
	IV	Intravenous	Route of administering fluid/ drugs into a vein
	IVI	Intravenous infusion	Fluid given via a vein, some-times shortened to IV
	O	Oral	By mouth
	SC	Subcutaneous	Route of injection into subcuta-neous tissue, below the dermis and epidermis layers of the skin

	Abbreviation	Term in full	Definition, common examples of use and notes
Gases	CO_2	Carbon dioxide	
	H	Hydrogen	
	N	Nitrogen	
	NO_2	Nitrous oxide	
	O_2	Oxygen	
Prescription frequencies (may also be written in capitals)	a.c.	Ante cibum	Before food
	b.d.	Bis die	Twice daily
	o.d.	Omni die	Once a day
	o.m.	Omne mane	In the morning (sometimes written *mané*)
	o.n.	Omne nocte	At night (sometimes written *nocté*)
	p.c.	Post cibum	After food
	p.r.n.	Pro re nata	As required
	q.d.s.	Quater die sumendum	Four times per day
	q.i.d.	Quater in die	Four times a day
	q.q.h.	Quaque quarta hora	Every 4 hours
	Stat.	Statim	Immediately
	t.d.s.	Ter die sumendum	Three times a day
	t.i.d.	Ter in die	Three times a day

Other abbreviations

£	pound (money)	
BNF	British National Formulary	
BSA	body surface area	Estimates of BSA may be more accurate than weight for calculating children's doses
cap.	capsule	
e/c	enteric coated	
FBC	fluid balance chart	
Hg	mercury	
H$_2$O	water	
hr	hour	
J	Joule	SI unit of energy – used in defibrillation
lb	pound (weight)	Imperial unit of weight (14 lbs = 1 stone)
min	minute	
NMC	Nursing and Midwifery Council	Statutory regulatory body for nurses and midwives in UK
oz	ounce	Imperial unit of weight (16 oz = 1 lb)
PICU	paediatric intensive care unit	
POM	prescription-only medicine	
SI	Système International d'Unités	International system of units – metric
Tab.	tablet	

Appendix B

Mathematical symbols

Symbol	Meaning
+	plus
−	minus
±	plus or minus
×	multiplied by
*	multiplied by
÷	divided by
/	divided by
=	equals
≈	approximately equal to
%	percent
∴	therefore
:	ratio of
>	greater than
<	less than (*hint: the symbol looks like L turned slightly clockwise*)
≤	less than or equal to
≥	more than or equal to

Appendix C

Glossary

See Appendix A for abbreviations.

Addition	The process of putting numbers together or combining them to find their *sum*.
Bolus	An amount given in one go. A one-off dose.
Centile	Centile charts show the distribution of a parameter within the population.
Decimal fraction	A decimal fraction is a decimal number that is less that 1, e.g. 0.75.
Denominator	The number below the line in a fraction.
Dialysis	Process by which blood is filtered to remove impurities.
Digit	One of the ten numerals from 0–9. A digit is given value by its place within a number.
Diluent or dilutent	A liquid used to reconstitute a powder to produce a solution, or a liquid used to dilute another to produce a weaker solution.
Displacement value	The increase in volume of a diluent when mixed with a powder.
Division	The process of separating an amount into a given number of equal parts. The result is the *quotient*.
Dose/dosage	The quantity of drug prescribed.
Dyscalculia	Combination of difficulties which primarily affect the learning of arithmetic facts and processing of numbers.
Dyslexia	Combination of difficulties that affect the processing and production of written language.
Enteric coated	Tablets with a special coating to protect the stomach lining.
Epidural	Refers to injection/infusion into the epidural space.
Equation	A statement of equality between two things.

Fraction	Part of a whole number, e.g. $\frac{3}{4}$.
Imperial measure	System of measures used prior to decimalization, e.g. pounds and ounces.
Intrathecal	Into the cerebrospinal fluid (CSF) within the dura.
Mixed number	A whole number and a fraction, e.g. $3\frac{1}{2}$.
Multiplication	Repeated addition. The number is added to itself a specific number of times resulting in the *product*.
Nomogram	A graphical representation of an equation.
Numerator	The number above the line in a fraction.
Reconstitution	Making up a solution by combining powder with a diluent.
Solute	Substance which dissolves in a solution.
Subtraction	The opposite of addition, resulting in their *difference*.
Top-heavy fraction	Fraction in which the numerator is greater than the denominator. May be changed to a mixed number.

Appendix D

Useful formulae

Oral medications

Tablets and capsules

$$\text{Number required} = \frac{\text{amount prescribed}}{\text{amount in each tablet or capsule}}$$

Liquids and suspensions

$$\text{Volume required} = \frac{\text{strength prescribed}}{\text{strength available}} \times \frac{\text{volume of stock}}{1}$$

Injections

$$\text{Volume required} = \frac{\text{strength prescribed}}{\text{strength available}} \times \frac{\text{volume of stock}}{1}$$

For tablets, liquids and injections, you can use the following formula, which can be remembered as 'NHS1'.

$$\frac{\text{What you Need}}{\text{What you Have}} \times \frac{\text{Stock amount}}{1}$$

Infusions

Automatic

$$\text{Rate (mL/hr)} = \frac{\text{Volume (mL)}}{\text{Time (hrs)}}$$

Manual

$$\text{Drip rate (drops/min)} = \frac{\text{drops/mL of the giving set} \times \text{volume}}{\text{number of hours to run} \times 60}$$

This can also be represented as the following formula, which can be remembered as a 'Very Tidy Drip Formula'.

$$\text{Drop rate (drops/min)} = \frac{\text{Volume (mL)}}{\text{Time (mins)}} \times \frac{\text{Drops Factors (drops/mL)}}{1}$$

Parenteral infusions

$$\text{Protocol time (hours)} = \frac{\text{volume of infusion}}{\text{flow rate}} + \text{break time}$$

Paediatric drugs

Dose required = body weight (kg) × recommended dose (mg/kg/day)

IV Flow Rates in mL/hr – VRT

The VRT figure below may be helpful in working with calculations involving flow rates.

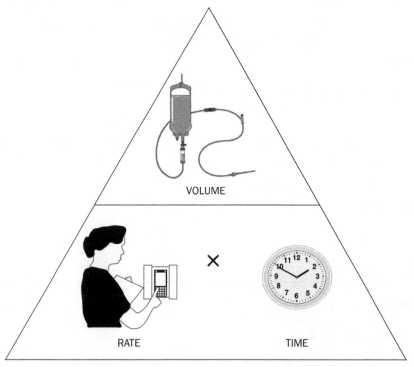

VOLUME

RATE × TIME

Source: Figure and text below about VRT is adapted from Karen Hudson, 2016. Reproduced with permission.

There are three elements to a flow rate calculation:

• **Volume** – the amount of fluid to be delivered
• **Rate** – the flow rate in mL/hr
• **Time** – the amount of time taken

Use the triangle by covering up the element that you want to work out. You will be left with the correct formula for your calculation.

Rate (mL/hr) = Volume (mL) ÷ Time (hrs)

Time (hrs) = Volume (mL) ÷ Rate (mL/hr)

Volume (mL) = Rate (mL/hr) × Time (hrs)

Remember – the fluid bag is high up!

The mnemonic **V**ery **R**arely **T**roubled may also help you to remember the formula.